NOT JUST WALKING

NOT JUST WALKING

✦

From Gifted Athlete to Quadriplegic—A Life of Multiple Sclerosis With the Help of True Love

Van E. Graef

iUniverse, Inc.

New York Lincoln Shanghai

NOT JUST WALKING
From Gifted Athlete to Quadriplegic—A Life of Multiple Sclerosis With the Help of True Love

Copyright © 2006 by Van E. Graef

iUniverse books may be ordered through booksellers or by contacting:

iUniverse
2021 Pine Lake Road, Suite 100
Lincoln, NE 68512
www.iuniverse.com
1-800-Authors (1-800-288-4677)

ISBN-13: 978-0-595-38133-3 (pbk)
ISBN-13: 978-0-595-82501-1 (ebk)
ISBN-10: 0-595-38133-2 (pbk)
ISBN-10: 0-595-82501-X (ebk)

Printed in the United States of America

Contents

INTRODUCTION

One day, I was doing what I did most days: sitting at home in my wheelchair, watching television. I'd been doing the same thing since 1998, when my wife and I sold the sports bar.

My youngest son, Tucker, bounced into the room with his bright blue eyes and childish grin. Then he plopped on the old couch and started watching a segment on Kelly's book club on Regis and Kelly with me. After a while, he said, "Hey, Dad, you should do that."

"Do what, Tuck?"

"Write a book. You've had a very interesting life. You can tell people about it."

Out of the mouths of babes, I thought. Even though Tucker is only twelve years old, he is pretty smart. At one point, I was having so much trouble picking up the mouse that I'd have to ask someone to give it to me. Tucker stopped by my computer one day and said, "You should get a cordless mouse." He was right, and it's because of him and his comments that I am writing this book and not just sitting in my chair watching TV.

Now don't get me wrong; I still do my share of TV watching. And I still have some problems using the computer and the microphone, so I do have some downtime. But Tucker's comments that day were just the push I needed to start working again.

◆　　◆　　◆

My son is right. I have had a very interesting life. The first thirty years could be a separate book, but the last twenty years or so have been the most interesting and informative. I certainly can't guarantee that reading about my life experiences will help anyone else, but maybe I can guide someone a little and prevent them from making the same mistakes. It might be entertaining to read about some of my experiences firsthand and see what I did. Many events in my life have been funny, and a few have been downright ridiculous. Others have been life-threatening dilemmas.

I always considered myself a completely normal person, at least physically. Sports came very easily for me. But the gradual changes caused by my disease, starting with the initial difficulty of moving, and progressing to being totally confined to a power wheelchair and unable to hold a pen or turn the pages of a book, have been devastating.

This is my story: early memories of being normal and active, then being diagnosed with a debilitating disease, and eventually coping and learning to keep a positive attitude through the worst of times. There were some bad times early in my life and, of course, some good times. My battle with multiple sclerosis has not been totally negative. Difficult at times, but not totally negative.

When I originally considered writing this book, I spoke with my oldest son, Kane. He said, "Whatever you do, tell all, and tell the truth." I agreed with him, but then I thought of Jerry Seinfeld. In one episode, when George was going to tell a girl that he loved her, Jerry said to George, "Are you sure of the return 'I love you?' Because if you're not sure, that's a big matzo ball out there."

Let me explain a little. The people who know me from my younger years are from New Jersey, and they know of my past. Then I moved to Colorado. Not being real proud of my first thirty years, I didn't tell a lot of people about my early life. Of course, the most important person in my life is my wife, Kathleen, and I did tell her everything when our relationship began. However, there are many friends and relatives who do not know the whole story.

I thought a lot about leaving out this part of my tale, but I decided that the people who didn't know me in the first thirty years would not judge me on something that happened a long time ago. I felt that they would judge me more on what they know of me now. I guess it's like finding out a good friend that you value and trust was a mass murderer early in his life. Maybe not that drastic, but you see what I mean. So, if you are a new friend or relative, please, if you decide to read my story (especially the first thirty years), remember me as the person I am now. Remember that your Kathleen has always known the whole story, and she still loves me. Thank you for understanding.

Not long after I decided to write this book, before I began the actual writing, I had a dream. I've often found that my dreams have helped me in life. This particular dream had to do with my work and people who worked for me. It began with me walking into a business and approaching a desk where there seemed to be a lot of activity. When I got to the desk, I recognized the person there. It was my friend and employee, Dee Dee Ridley.

"How far have you gotten on the job?" I asked.

Dee Dee smiled. "It's all done."

"You guys must have really been hustling."

"We are not just walking around here," Dee Dee joyfully proclaimed.

I had the title to my book. After all, my life is certainly more about other things than it is about not walking. It has been more than ten years since I could hold a pen and write. Typing was totally out of the question. I tried using a tape recorder to tell my story, but it just wasn't working. I would forget where I was and get sidetracked, even more than I do now.

One day, while out on the Internet, I noticed an advertisement for a voice recognition system that said you could talk to your computer, and it would type what you had said. I was a little leery of the idea, but I really wanted to see if it would work. So, I ordered the system, and in a week or so it arrived. I couldn't wait to start training it to recognize my voice and speech pattern.

The package contained articles and stories to read that would train the system. I read one whole story and thought I would finish the rest of the training the next day. But when I tried to retrieve the training stories, they were gone. So I just began using the program to see if it would work. After just one training session, it would type, but not anything I had said. I noticed the longer I spoke into it, the better the typing got. So, I decided to start this book. As far as a word processing program, all I had was Microsoft WordPad, but I started off anyway.

I quickly realized that I needed a better program, so I purchased Microsoft Works. My very pretty sister-in-law, Lynne, said that she wanted to read what I had done and that she would correct it.

The first few pages were very funny and quite entertaining. She read them, laughed, and corrected them. She said, "Whatever you do, do not destroy these pages. They will tell the story of how you wrote this book." I am including the first few pages of the original manuscript just so you can see what I am talking about. In the long run, this would make a great commercial for the makers of the voice recognition program. It's amazing that I got the book completed with just that small amount of training.

I would like to thank Dragon Systems for their program and help. Without you and the Dragon Systems Point and Speak for Dummies booklet, there would be no book, and my story would never be told. Thank you. Hey, maybe there's some money to be made here!

I always thought that maybe I could write a book. Then I would think, Who am I to think I could write a book? I was a poor to average student. I only went to school so I could play sports. My goal in college was to become a physical education teacher. People said, "Ha ha, you're dumb." Fortunately, I eventually studied banking.

Now I guess I have something to say and the time to say it. One day, my wife Kathleen and I were talking to our neighbors, Michale and Joyce. I met Joyce at the mall many moons ago. She is a manager at Wal-Mart. I have the utmost respect for Michale. He was a big deal in the Air Force before he retired. They have been really great neighbors, and I know Kathleen would not trade them for anyone.

Kathleen had mentioned to Michale that I had started writing a book. Michale said, "What would you have to say that I would want to read?" That question stayed with me for a long time.

Kathleen and I talked about the book often, but I never did anything about it until Tucker's comments during that TV program. I thought to myself, <u>Why not? If it's not any good, who cares? Just maybe somebody will want to hear what I have to say. And, maybe, someone might learn something. Or just be entertained</u>.

◆   ◆   ◆

As a final note, I wanted to talk a little about my experiences with the ladies. Fortunately, I did learn something from each and every one of my relationships. I feel each experience has made me a better person. I always tell my wife I had to go through a lot of shit to become the person I've become. She's not happy about me talking about this, but I think it's important for my readers to know a person can change.

It's like the old Willie Nelson song, <u>To All The Girls I've Loved Before</u>. When I was much younger, I did most of my thinking with something other than my brain, if you know what I mean. For some reason, I had the reputation of being a ladies' man. Sometimes I felt if I didn't sleep with some girl, my peers would wonder what was wrong. I didn't always treat those girls fairly, and I wasn't always truthful. <u>Please accept my apologies</u>.

CHAPTER 1
Jersey Boy
The Beginning

I have decided to begin at the beginning, that's the best place as any. The two parts of my life, that would be before my diagnosis with multiple sclerosis and then after being diagnosed. Everything that happened in my early life, the girls, my relatives, sports, work and all the bad decisions I made did prepare me for dealing with the debilitating disease. Multiple sclerosis [MS] is weird. It treats everyone a little different. The only experience I can relate to is my own. I remember being diagnosed and saying, "I will never be in a wheelchair." I fought the disease hard only to realize that you can not fight this disease. Fighting only makes the disease take over. Once I realized that you cannot fight it and you have to deal with what the disease gives or takes from you, I was able to cope. When I finally did have to go to a wheelchair, it wasn't all that bad. Boxers fight and sufferers deal with what they get.

I wouldn't wish this disease on my worst enemy. However, you can not be bitter. That gets you nowhere. A bitter person is tough to be around. Isn't it better to have a positive attitude? A positive attitude helps you to manage no matter what you are dealt.

I have seen pictures of my mother and father together when they were young. They looked like they belonged together. My mother was a cute little thing. She was a cheerleader type. My father was in his

Marine uniform, five feet eleven inches tall, well built and handsome, from what I understand.

My brother is George Milton Graef, III. He is four years older, and was born when my father was in the Marines fighting the war. My mother named him after my father, but from the day he was born she called him Chip. That had something to do with a movie she was watching around the time he was born. We still call him Chip today.

When I was born, my father, my mother, and my brother were living in an old farmhouse not far from Plainfield, New Jersey, in a little town called Green Brook. They called the house The Apple Tree House and my father, a carpenter, had great plans to fix it up. I don't remember anything about the house, but I have seen pictures, especially one of me with a big bandage on my right hand. I had touched the wood-burning stove, and the burn must have been pretty bad. Throughout my life, I've done routine things left-handed, such as writing, combing my hair, and brushing my teeth. The important things, like throwing and batting, I did right-handed.

At such a young age, I didn't know that my parents were having marital difficulties. The next thing I remember is that my mother, my brother, and I were living in an apartment in a big complex in Bound Brook, New Jersey.

My mother worked as a secretary to a vice president of a large manufacturing company in a neighboring town. After high school, she had attended a secretarial school in New York City. Not only was she a fast typist, but she also took shorthand.

I guess she made pretty good money. We had a car and clothes on our backs, and we weren't hungry all the time. We didn't see my father much. I remember getting dressed and sitting on the steps of the apartment, waiting. I didn't care one way or the other, but Chip would be excited. Dad never showed up.

Our father also never gave our mother any money. I remember her telling me that she had taken him to court to get the back child support he owed her. Well, she didn't get any money from him, but they lowered his monthly payment. He never paid that either.

I also remember sitting in the apartment with all the lights out. My mother would whisper, "Let's pretend we're not home." She would shush us, and then after a knock at the door, we would wait for the bill collector to leave. Then it would be just the three of us again.

There was a brook not far from the apartment complex. As far back as I can remember, whenever I got the chance, I headed to the brook with my fishing rod. My special spot was at a point in the brook where a large tree had fallen and washed downstream. The roots were still attached to the base of the tree and had dug a deep hole where it stopped. I would catch catfish, sunfish, suckers, and several types of minnows. I loved that place and spent a lot of time there trying to out-smart the fish.

◆   ◆   ◆

When I was about four years old, my mother hired a young girl to take care of me for the summer. She wasn't a nice girl, and wouldn't let me go outside the whole summer. She also abused me sexually. She was always touching my penis. I remember lying on the bed with no clothes on. One day she took a shiny new nail and inserted it into the opening of my penis. I also remember her opening the cat's mouth and inserting my penis in it. Of course, the cat bit me, and I still have the scar today. The sitter threatened me, so I never told my mother. I am sure that the episodes from that summer caused many of my adult hang-ups.

My brother usually ignored the sitter and got to do anything he wanted. But one day she made him mad, and he started throwing things at her. That was the beginning of the end for her. When we told our mother what had been going on, she got rid of the girl, and I was on my own. Years later, my mother told me that the girl had become a teacher. It figures.

◆   ◆   ◆

Every summer we spent our vacation in North Jersey. My mother's parents had a cabin on Highland Lakes. I was told that it had cost $1500 to build in the 1940s. The cabin was great. It had electricity, but no heat, except for a large fireplace that would take the chill off the night. The cabin had two large bedrooms, a bath, a small kitchen, a large living area, and a screened porch. Being right on the lake, the place had a dock and a rowboat. At an early age, I learned to row the boat. I often went out alone and fished.

The bedroom where my brother and I slept had bunk beds and one single bed. The wall in the bedroom did not reach the ceiling, and from the top bunk we could see into the large room where the fireplace was.

There was also a window in the bedroom that looked out toward the lake. During the summer that window stayed open, and in the morning we could hear the lake gently lapping against the side of the wooden rowboat. I still hear it in my memory. Whenever I heard that sound, I knew it was time to go fishing.

Several members of my maternal grandmother's family had cabins at Highland Lake, too. My grandmother's brother and sister had the cabin right next to ours. The Sedlock family lived on the other side, and Andy Sedlock was like the law at the lake. He also acted as the game warden, probably because the Sedlocks lived at the lake all year long.

Young John Sedlock was my age. We were inseparable the whole vacation time, and he taught me a lot about the lake and about fishing. His older sister married one of my mother's cousins, and I always referred to John as my cousin.

When I was in junior high, my grandparents retired, moved to Florida, and sold the lake house. They offered to sell it to anyone in the family first, but no one took them up on it. I know my mother would have loved to buy it, but she couldn't afford it. Still, once I got my driver's license, I would drive to the lake to visit John and do a little fishing.

During the last trip my wife and I made to New Jersey, we took a ride to the lake. Some things had changed, but most were the same. There was no one I knew there at the time, but it was nice to see the old cabin and the lake. If I ever had a lot of money, I would like to buy the cabin. It's probably worth a small fortune now.

◆   ◆   ◆

During the school year, when my mother would come home from work, she would throw the ball to my brother and me. It must have done some good. Chip was only eight when he tried out for Little League, and he made the team. In fact, the very first game he played, he pitched a no-hitter. That's pretty good for an eight-year-old pitching against nine-, ten-, eleven-, and twelve-year-olds. The Little League field was on the way to the brook, so I would stop by every game and watch him.

I couldn't wait until I turned eight to try out for the Little League team. In those days, the tryouts lasted two days, and they started on Saturday. Unfortunately, that year, it was also the first day of trout season. I went fishing. I showed up the second day, but I guess they thought I would rather fish than play ball. I didn't make the team I wanted, and they put me on a team in the minor leagues. We didn't have uniforms, just t-shirts and caps, and the field was about a half-mile away from home. It just wasn't the same.

My brother was always tall and well-proportioned, and I was plump. Chip teased me about being chunky, and told everyone I wore husky-sized jeans. I would never wear shorts or short-sleeved shirts in my younger days. Then, during the summer of my thirteenth year, I grew up instead of out, and when school started, no one recognized me.

Late that summer, my mother started dating this guy named George. He was a small man, and he walked with a pretty bad limp. I can't remember why. Whenever he talked, there always seemed to be a little spit in the corner of his mouth. George chain-smoked, about five packs a day, and he couldn't quit. It eventually killed him. He worked in New York City as an import/export agent, and commuted to the city by train. Poppa George, as I called him, always wore bow ties. He also had some kind of skin problem. His skin was flaky and he had bad dandruff, but going to the doctor never seemed to help.

Chip and I thought George had some money, but we couldn't be sure. He had a son named Skip from his first marriage. Skip would show up every other weekend, and the three of us boys got along okay.

Working in the city, Poppa George often got Yankees tickets. He would take my brother and me to Yankee Stadium pretty regularly. I remember the very first time I saw the field. It was green and beautiful, with sparkling white bases and a brown infield. The advertising around the outfield was bright and colorful. The sight was something a young baseball fan would always remember.

From 1957 to 1960, the Yankees had some great players: Mickey Mantle in center field, Tony Kubek at short, Bobby Richardson at second, Clete Boyer at third, Moose Skowron at first, Elston Howard catching, and Whitey Ford pitching. When I was in junior high, a friend and I would skip school and grab a bus or train to New York City to watch the Yankees play. A few years later, when I was in high school, the whole baseball team went to Yankee Stadium. The basketball team got to go to the National Invitational Tournament at the old Madison Square Garden before it was rebuilt in a new location.

The last time I was at Yankee Stadium was in 1978. I had a friend who said he had good tickets to the game. I really didn't take him very seriously, but when we got to the stadium, the seats were on the Yankee's dugout. They were great seats, and it was a great game.

◆   ◆   ◆

Before Chip and I knew it, our mother and George were married, and we were moving to the rival town of Somerville. We moved into another large apartment complex. Of course, my brother and I transferred to the local public school, and had no problem making new friends.

I got along with George pretty well, but my brother had a real problem with him. Chip was thirteen years old by then, and he towered over George. He just did not like the man at all, which made for some tense family moments.

As spring approached, Somerville had Little League tryouts, too. I was now nine years old, the tryouts weren't on the first day of trout season, and I made a team.

But at home, my mother and George were having some problems. My brother and I went skating every Saturday night, and one evening George picked us up at the roller rink and drove us home. He didn't come into the apartment with us, which we thought was a little strange. When we got inside, Mom was sitting in the dark. When Chip turned on the light, our mother was on the couch, crying. As she lifted her head, we saw blood trickling from the corner of her mouth. She and George had gotten into a fight, and he'd popped her one. Needless to say, the three of us left that night.

We eventually moved into the same old complex in Somerville, and it was just the three of us again. Our mother and George had only been married for about a year. She changed her name back to Graef, just so she would have our last name and not cause any undue confusion.

Chip and I did okay in school. We had really gotten into sports. My brother, being older, had more chances to play different sports in junior high and high school. Until I got into junior high, I had only had Little League baseball. Once I got into junior high, like my brother, I started playing football and basketball, too.

Chip didn't excel in basketball, so it was the only game I could ever beat him in. I didn't pick up a basketball until I was nine years old, but I really enjoyed the game once I got started. And if you really enjoy doing something, practicing is a pleasure. By the time I got to junior high, I had gotten pretty good. I especially enjoyed playing in front of a crowd.

About this time, we moved from the apartment complex to a duplex on the east end of town. Chip's friend's parents owned it. It was a nice place, and we each had our own room, which was a first. Unfortunately, we were only there for a year before Mel's parents sold it. We then moved to the south end of town, into a house right next to the cemetery. It had a long, paved driveway and an empty lot on the opposite side.

Chip and I utilized the cemetery grounds and the empty lot to practice. In the cemetery, it was difficult to run a pass pattern without charging into the head stones, but in the empty lot we would punt the football back and forth for hours. We both became punters on our football teams.

We lived on the bottom floor of the house and the landlords, the Potters, lived upstairs. Mr. Potter had been the Fire Chief, and drove the garbage truck for the town. This came in handy when my brother needed to earn money for school. I think Mr. Potter also helped me get a job with the town the summer before I went to college.

Somerville was the town where my father grew up. Actually, when I got to high school, there were still two teachers who'd been there when my father went to school. One of the teachers was a French teacher. The other, Sam Yohn, taught physical education and had coached me in track. He was the athletic director when I went to school, and he gave an award every year for the senior with the most athletic ability. I'm proud to say I won it my senior year.

CHAPTER 2
Mom and The Male Parental Unit

Mom. What a great lady. She was sort of petite. I guess she was good looking, but everyone thinks their own mother is pretty. I remember once when my brother and I were in high school, he had either said or done something she didn't like, and my mother punched him on the arm. Of course, it didn't hurt Chip, but Mom hurt her wrist. She acted as both our mother and our father, and she really took good care of us.

Mom smoked most of her life, and she enjoyed a beer or three. Cigarettes were not good to her. Later in life she had terrible emphysema and was on oxygen all the time.

My mother's parents, Ruth Edwards and William Van Blarcom, were religious folks. Grandma was a small person like our mother, and just as cute as a bug's ear. Grandpa, on the other hand, was six feet five inches tall. He didn't need to yell. He only had to look at you, and you knew you were in trouble.

My grandparents had three children, Lois Ruth, William Joseph, and Philip Lewis. Philip, the youngest, was born about twenty years after mom. He isn't much older than my brother Chip.

Our mother and her brothers were born and raised in Franklin, New Jersey. Franklin is in northern New Jersey, in Sussex County. From there, they moved to Jersey City and eventually to Bound Brook. Grandpa was the postmaster on the train, and Grandma was a homemaker. People called Grandpa Mr. Van. We had a close relationship with our mother's parents, and Mom, Chip, and I spent all our holidays at their house.

Is it a wonder that my first name is Van? My middle name is Edwards. My whole name is a collection of last names.

Lois Ruth, our mother, graduated from Bound Brook High School. She was a cheerleader and very smart. But she must have taken a lot of sick days, because in her yearbook it said, "An occasional day off breaks up the monotony."

After secretarial school in New York City, Mom got a job at Johns Manville Corp. She was secretary to one of the vice presidents in the research department. Johns Manville makes transit pipe and various roofing materials. The factory and the research center were located in Manville, which is just west of Bound Brook. It seemed as though nearly everyone in the family worked there at one time or another.

As my mother told this story, she was at a party one night and there was this handsome guy there. After they talked for a while, he asked her out. They dated for some time, but my mother refused to give up her virtue. Mom always said that was why our father finally gave in and married her. After they got married, they moved in with my mother's parents.

My mother was very intelligent. When you needed a word spelled, she could do it. She was always reading or doing a crossword puzzle. I could call her anytime I needed an answer. To this day, if I am stumped on something, my first thought is to call her, even though she passed away in February 1997.

◆   ◆   ◆

Around 1965, my mother met a guy that she had known in high school. Art was a big shot in the insurance industry. He also had his private pilot's license. He would take my mother on short flights to have dinner at fancy restaurants on the east coast.

Art didn't bother with my brother and me, but he and Mom were always together. They had been seeing each other for long enough that I'm sure there'd been talk of a wedding. We knew our mother was very much in love. Art was the first guy she had been interested in since the end of her second marriage in 1960. Art treated my mother well and also seemed to be in love.

After about a year, out of the blue, Art broke the relationship off. My mother was devastated. She went to the doctor, who sent her to New Jersey Psychiatric Institute in Skillman, New Jersey. Before long, the doctors there realized that she shouldn't be institutionalized. Mom was heartbroken, and a little depressed, but certainly not crazy or mentally deranged. She did seem to benefit from the month's rest, though. We never heard from Art again.

◆　　　◆　　　◆

Good old Dad was born in Somerville in January of 1915. Our grandparents, George Milton Graef, Sr., and Alvina McCubbin Graef, had moved to Somerville from Baltimore. They had three children: Elsie, Richard and George, Jr. Grandpa Graef worked as an accountant at Johns Manville.

I have seen pictures of Grandpa and Grandma Graef. Grandpa was a thin man with a big mustache. Grandma was on the plump side. I guess my father, who was younger than his siblings, took after his father. We never had a close relationship with our paternal grandparents, because they passed away either before I was born or shortly thereafter.

My father, George Jr., attended Somerville High School. He told me that he quit school a month before graduation because he was going to fail anyway. After quitting school, he joined the family ranks and went to work for Johns Manville.

I guess the old man was pretty handsome. He had thick brown hair that he wore pretty short, but not cut in a butch. Dad had the palest blue eyes. Chip has those same blue eyes. When he worked for Johns Manville, they asked him to do some promotional photos, which I still have.

Since our father and mother were not bad looking people, my brother and I had a head start in the looks department. We both were voted best looking in our senior class polls.

I didn't know until I got into high school that our father still held a track record for the 220. We hadn't seen him much during this time, but we found out that he was quite an athlete. So, Chip and I also had a head start in the athletic department. To say the least, our life was sports, sports, and more sports.

I learned years later that our father had been invited to run in the Penn relays in the 1930s, which was essentially a tryout for the U.S. Olympic team. The Olympics were not as big then as they are today, and our father told me he didn't go because he had something better to do that day. Knowing him, I'm sure it had to do with either a woman or alcohol.

The Olympics were held in Germany, and it was the year Jesse Owens did so well. The day our father told me this story, we were out fishing on Swartzwood Lake. When it was just the two of us, in a boat in the middle of the lake, he would talk about his past.

As a change of life baby, our father was much younger than his siblings. I think, because of his parents' age, that he may have become a little hard to handle. I know he spent some of his youth at a place called Toleman's Pond, in Keene, New Hampshire. He took me there once when I was about twelve. He told me how he had skied to and from school, and how he had fished the pond. While we were there, I fished the pond and caught some nice small-mouth bass. He had a good time visiting old friends while we were there.

My father also told me once that while he was in high school, he had dated a teacher. I suppose it's possible. Nowadays teachers date students all the time. But in the late 1930s? Anyway, he said she got pregnant, and he offered to marry her, but she refused, and left Somerville to get an abortion.

After my mother and he were divorced, he married a lady he worked with named Lindy. I always liked her, but Chip didn't like her at all. While Lindy was very smart, she wasn't a real attractive person. My brother used to call her the old witch. Are you seeing a theme here with my brother? Right. He didn't like anyone.

Lindy taught piano and loved the outdoors and nature. She could be a real fanatic. I always thought that Lindy was mad at me for digging up worms and using them to catch fish.

One time I asked my father why he didn't stay with Mom. He told me that my mother came to him to try to reconcile, but he told her he'd already made a commitment to Lindy. That seemed to be his excuse for not supporting us or seeing us regularly.

Once, when my brother found out the old man was having financial difficulties, he offered to set him and Lindy up in Colorado. Chip said that he would rent them an apartment close by, and we would both take care of them financially. My father declined the offer, saying he had to stay in Florida, because Lindy's sister was sick and in bad shape. Chip never contacted him again.

I'm sure that Lindy knew of my father's running around. He told me that Lindy had some sort of problem with her sexual parts, as if that justified his actions.

My father used to come and see me play sports at the strangest locations. Of course, I found out later that watching me play wasn't the only reason he would come to town. There was also the camp nurse, and who knows who else. My mother told me that he would stop and visit her two or three times a year when she was living alone, and he wasn't there just to say hello.

When my father was having problems in Florida, my brother called the church, and they sent people out to help. Being a good Methodist, he was offered a job setting up a camp in North Jersey. He was in charge of the whole place. He did carpentry work, cooking, and nearly everything else that needed to be done. I visited the camp quite often, once I was driving. It was located in a little town called Swartzwood. There was a nice lake there, of course, which I fished quite often. There was also a pond and a stream at the camp, which grew quite large and hosted lots of kids. The Methodist church built a house on the campgrounds for my father and Lindy. My father worked there for about twenty years before he retired.

I don't know what else to say about my father. He did like the ladies, and he really enjoyed a cocktail or two or three every day. As he aged, his athletic shape went to pot, literally. I don't know if it was from all the beer, but he developed quite a large belly. When my brother and I were younger, we always said we would never look like that when we got older. Still, my brother did get pretty big. He didn't miss many meals.

Dad was a good-hearted guy who used to laugh a lot and really enjoyed cooking. As a matter of fact, he owned two restaurants at one point in his life. He opened a rotisserie shop and cooked chickens in the window. I was about ten years old at the time. It may have been the very first take-out. But people just weren't ready for that yet in the 1950s. My father could've been the first Colonel Sanders, but he was just a little ahead of his time.

The second restaurant was a truck stop along the busiest highway in the county. Unfortunately, they had started building a new interstate just north of his restaurant. So as soon as that new interstate opened, it closed my father's restaurant. That was the last attempt he made at owning a restaurant, but he did a lot of cooking for the kids at the Methodist camp called Aldersgate.

Mom told me once that when my father was young, he wanted to become a singer. She said he took lessons, and she used to go with him. My mother said it was very painful to listen to my father sing. I have sat next to him in church, and I can attest that he sings loud and off-key.

CHAPTER 3
Somerville, New Jersey

Let me tell you a little bit about the town of Somerville, population 12,400. Main Street was great for cruising during our high school years. Somerville is bordered on the north by Highway 22 and on the south by the Raritan River, which I used to fish a lot. It was pretty dirty, with a lot of carp and suckers. But upstream it flows a little faster and used to be stocked with trout. It actually runs all the way to the Atlantic Ocean. To the west of town is Highway 206 and the town of Raritan.

Peters Brook runs through the middle of town and eventually flows into the Raritan River. I used to fish it a lot, and even caught trout in it, along with catfish, suckers, sunfish, chubs, and minnows. It was a pretty good little fishing hole, and it was close by. I once saw a lamprey eel swimming around. They were pretty common in the Raritan River. During the winters the brook would freeze over, and we would skate on it.

One of the best places to fish was Clay Hole, located just west of town, behind the state trooper barracks. Our fishing trips to Clay Hole were routinely interrupted by state troopers checking on us to make sure we weren't doing anything illegal.

Somerville was a great little town to grow up in. You could get anywhere in town on foot. Somerville is the county seat for Somerset County. When I was growing up, Somerville's favorite son was Lee Van Cleef, the actor. He was pretty famous, and he starred in <u>The Good, The Bad, and The Ugly</u> and <u>Who Shot Liberty Valance,</u> plus a whole lot of cowboy films. When he came to town, he was known to drink a bit. Supposedly, one time he got drunk and drove his car across the courthouse lawn, making the powers-to-be very unhappy. But being who he was, he didn't get into any trouble. He used to come to Somerville and hang out at the Gateway Inn. Just prior to his passing, he was visiting Somerville and was at the Gateway. A friend of mine happened to be at the bar at the same time. My friend told me that he got to talk to Mr. Van Cleef and the beautiful girl who was with him. My friend said he was just a regular guy.

One of Somerville's claims to fame is that George Washington slept there at the Wallace house. Somerville also has an annual bicycle race through town called the Tour de Somerville, which was started by a local bicycle shop owner named Pop Kugler. Because his son and the first winner of the race were both killed in World War II, it is named the Kugler Anderson Tour de Somerville.

Raritan, the town just west of Somerville, was the home of World War II Medal of Honor winner John Basilone. They erected a big statue of him just west of town. After he had won the Medal of Honor, he was selling war bonds, but he wasn't happy, so he went back to the war and was killed at Iwo Jima.

My Uncle Bill was also a marine. All marines know of Manila John Basilone. My Uncle Bill had never met John Basilone, but he told me that when he was running onto the beach at Iwo Jima, he saw John's name on a toe tag on a body on the beach.

Many families just stay in Somerville. Most of my friends are still living there. When I was going to school, the town really supported the school's athletes and athletic programs. All the storeowners knew you by your first name if you played football. The Pioneer Club, the high school booster club, would have pictures taken of the starters on the football team every year and would post them in the downtown stores. At the end of the season, they would give them to us. At one point, I had two of my pictures, but I gave them to girls and never got them back.

CHAPTER 4
S H S—The Glory Days

When I was a freshman in high school, my brother was a senior. It was pretty cool, because all the older girls knew me. The coaches also knew who I was because of my brother.

The night of my freshman dance, I had a date with another freshman named Jill Neumann. Remember that name. We had a nice time at the dance, and I walked her home. I don't even recall getting a kiss. As I was walking home from Jill's house, an old Chevy pulled up with a bunch of my brother's friends in it. They asked me if I wanted to go to a party where my brother was. Of course I said yes. The party was pretty cool. All the varsity football players were there. There was also some beer, which we were allowed to drink as long as we spent the night. One of my brother's friends came walking in with a girl and said, "Give Van a big kiss," and she did. Her name was Penny Nuss. She was a sophomore and also a cheerleader. She was a real cute blonde. It was the beginning of a beautiful relationship. We went together for three years. We had a lot of fun together. I learned a lot from her about girls and life in general.

◆   ◆   ◆

The summer before my senior year, my brother said to me, "You know, your senior year you should be free and have fun." Penny had already graduated and was working in a dentist's office. Well, I always listened to my brother, so I broke up with her. Don't get me wrong.

17

There were other girls before Penny. I guess I was taking after my father. I did like the ladies and at the beer parties, I learned I liked the booze, too.

I sure enjoyed sports, but in order to play, you had to pass your classes. Not being the best student, I really had to work hard.

When I was a sophomore, I quit the football team. I just didn't like the practices, and I was up against juniors and seniors. I guess the competition was getting to me. I started hanging around some guys who were not a very good influence, and we broke into a house. I guess my brother found out about it, and he told me that if I didn't go back to football, he would kick my ass. Knowing my brother was not kidding, I went back to the coach and asked if I could rejoin the team. The coach let me back on the team since I had only quit for about two weeks. After rejoining the team, I settled down and got back to work.

In football, I loved playing in the games, but practices were not a lot of fun. I was a receiver and enjoyed catching the ball. We ran the old T formation. The ends had to block a lot, and we didn't do much passing.

After all that practicing with my brother through the years, I was pretty damn good. Add in all the parties and fun times we had just because we were on the football team, and you know we had a lot of friends. After we'd gone through all the football nonsense together, some of them were very close friends.

Being on the football team definitely had its benefits. It's like instant popularity, and you feel as though you have done things that other people could not do. Students having parties always invited the football team. They knew that we would go to New York and buy beer and keep the peace if any rowdies showed up at the party.

During one of our many road trips to Staten Island to buy liquor for a party, four of us—Stan Jackowky, John Parks, Mark Manara, and me—jumped into Stanley's Ford Falcon (a sweet ride called Midnight Passion—powder blue with blue interior lights) and headed east. The rule was that no one could drink any liquor until we got to the party.

We purchased several cases of beer and a couple of specialty drinks that the girls liked. Their favorite was Tango, a pre-made screwdriver in a quart bottle. Mark and I sat in the front with Stan, and John sat in the back with the liquor.

Putting John in the back with the liquor was our first mistake. John Parks was an offensive guard on the football team and catcher on the baseball team. He had done some weightlifting and was very muscular. He was also a big joker and wasn't scared of anything.

It was quiet in the back seat. I happened to glance back at John, and he had the Tango bottle lifted to his mouth and was taking the last swallow. We all screamed at him and recited the rule.

John had a pivot tooth in the front of his mouth. He started to scream that he had lost his tooth and began looking for it. He became very upset when he couldn't find it. He said his parents were going to kill him because the tooth was expensive, and it wasn't the first one he had lost.

We got to the party and started to party ourselves. Then I saw John running out the front door. I didn't think much of his behavior; that was the way John was. When I saw him again, he was inserting the tooth into his mouth. We were all happy for him. It turned out that the nasty Tango had gotten to him and he had gone outside to puke...thus finding his tooth. He could have washed it off first. That was Parksey.

John was a year behind me in school. I thought he was not the brightest bulb in the package at the time, but he showed me. After graduation, he went to Salem college, the same college I was attending, but a year after I had left. He, too, was a physical education major. He also played football, but instead of a lineman he was a fullback.

After he received his teaching degree, he realized that he hated teaching, so he came back to Somerville and lived with Bob, Winks, and me for a while. He did have a tryout with the New York Jets, but didn't make the team. Not knowing what to do next, John decided to go back to school and get his doctorate in chiropractic medicine. Who would have thought: <u>Dr. Parks</u>?

◆   ◆   ◆

Throughout high school, I remember everybody smoking. Some of the greatest athletes Somerville has ever known smoked. Back then it wasn't a big deal like it is today. Most of my brother's teammates smoked, and there were a few of us that smoked on my team. Some of the coaches smoked, too.

The summer before my senior year, one of my friends, Ralph Petrill, got caught buying cigarettes. Ralph was probably the best lineman Somerville had ever seen, but he got kicked off the football team.

I guess they were trying to make an example of him. Ralph was an okay student, and his parents were not wealthy. He knew he would need a football scholarship to go to college. He made the decision to go live with his aunt in Hazleton, Pennsylvania, to play his senior year. He did play and got his scholarship. Afterward, he told me that the football was much better in Pennsylvania.

I always felt bad that we hadn't stood up for Ralph, but we were all in the same situation. We needed to play for any chance of a scholarship. So we probably had one of the worst seasons in Somerville's football history, at least as far as win/loss records go.

The last time we visited New Jersey on the way back to Colorado we stopped in Hazleton, Pennsylvania. Ralph owns a sports bar in town. So we stopped and had a drink or two and visited with Ralph.

Whenever my family goes back to New Jersey, we try to see as many friends as we can. My best friend during high school was Mark Manara. We still stay in touch, and he still lives in Somerville. Mark is a great guy. We sure had a lot of fun, not only during high school, but also in later years.

◆   ◆   ◆

When my mother, brother and I first moved to Somerville, I would go to the high school games, so I knew the guys that played well before me. By the time I became a senior, some of these guys were teachers, which was pretty cool.

After football season came basketball, and after basketball came baseball. It was the thing to do in the spring and summer. I enjoyed playing the outfield but also did some pitching. With all the Little League play, by the time I got to high school, the game came pretty naturally.

During the summers we played pony league, and the summer I was fifteen, I was asked to play in the semi-pro league. The other players were in college, or had played professionally at one time. We kept our amateur status as long as we weren't paid to play. The only thing that I ever received was a hot dog or two.

One Sunday morning, the coach called me to ask if my brother would like to pitch. My brother had played for the Houston Astros in the minor leagues for several years, but he had hurt his arm, was at home, and hadn't signed with any team yet.

I asked Chip if he would pitch in the game and he said he would. That was the only baseball game we ever played together. I played center field and he pitched. I think we won, but my brother hurt his arm again. I didn't know it, but he'd gotten an offer to play with the Detroit Tigers. He'd agreed to play with their minor league team in Canada, but he hadn't signed the contract yet. But Chip didn't go to Canada, because he decided to go back to college.

As I said, I saw my brother's first no-hitter in Little League. I also watched him pitch a no-hitter in high school. It was impressive. During that game the centerfielder, John Gara, made an unbelievable shoe-string catch to preserve my brother's no-hitter. Chip's sophomore year, I watched him pitch in the state finals. He started the game, but when he ran into a little trouble, the coach brought in someone else to pitch, and my brother moved to left field. Then he was brought back as pitcher to clean up the game. Not only that, but the shortstop, Joe Liss, stroked a homerun to right center field for the win.

John Gara went on to college in Pennsylvania, and became a physical education teacher at a nearby high school. John's younger brother, Ron, was the quarterback during my senior year. He also played basketball and baseball.

Joe Liss graduated, then signed to play baseball for the Philadelphia Phillies, where he joined another Somerville graduate, Fireball Freddie Wenz. Joe was eventually traded to the Minnesota Twins. Now, Joe and his son run a baseball camp in Florida.

I met a scout from the Chicago White Sox when I was a junior in high school. I guess he was there to look at someone else, but I had a good game. The coach stopped him from talking to me by telling him I was only a junior. The scout said he would see me next year. I had a pretty good senior year, but I never saw him again.

I hope my readers won't think I'm full of hogwash for writing about this. I was All-County in football, basketball, and baseball, too. I've included some news articles and photos, to prove I'm not just blowing smoke.

Back in 1966, in the middle of football season my senior year, the coach told the receivers we weren't trying our hardest to catch passes, and he wanted us to dive after more balls. Later that day, when we were running pass patterns in the end zone, the quarterback threw a pass just out of my reach. Remembering what the coach had said, I dove to catch the ball.

Unfortunately, I dove right into the goal post and knocked myself out. Still, I continued diving for passes during our next game. I think I dove several times that game, but we still lost.

That game was played Saturday afternoon. On Sunday morning, my friend Mark Manara came over to my house and said, "I don't know if we'll be able to live with Van after I show him what I have."

He showed us a picture of me diving for the ball, completely stretched out, with the ball just touching my fingertips. He had cut it out of a local newspaper. I think every athlete has a picture he is most proud of, and that is mine.

One of the basketball games I remember most was played against our cross-town rival, Immaculata, a Catholic high school. We were at their gym and I had one of those games a lot of athletes dream of having. I was in the zone. It was almost like being in a dream. It was just one of those games where I could do no wrong offensively. I've said I felt like I could have kicked the ball into the basket.

I remember taking a jump shot from the corner and having two guys leaping in my face, trying to block my shot. When I let the ball go, I couldn't even see the basket. But I knew the ball went into the basket when the crowd roared.

Unfortunately, there are offensive and defensive parts to the game. Defensively, I had gotten into foul trouble quite early, so the coach took me out of the game for a while. After all was said and done, I had scored thirty points and had four fouls. We won the game, but if I hadn't had the foul problem, I am sure I could have broken the school record for most points in one game. I think the record at that time was 42.

One of my friends was the manager of the football team. He was a year ahead of me, and his name was Richard Panone. His parents had a house on Lake Hopatcong. It wasn't just a cabin; it was better than most people's homes. Rich had invited us to the lake house every once in a while, but it soon became a Friday night ritual. Our friend, Louis Strong, would pick up a couple of cases of beer. Louie was a year older and had a car, an old black Chrysler with a pushbutton transmission. That car could fly.

Now remember, I was still in high school, and Louie was a year ahead of me. It was a state law that you had to be twenty-one to buy or drink alcohol. Louie would put a pair of dark glasses on and visit a bar in a small town just west of Somerville. He played tackle on the foot-ball team and was a big guy, so he got away with it.

So every Friday night, Louie, Mark Manara, Rich and I would party at the lake. Rich's parents didn't show up until sometime Saturday, and we had the whole place to ourselves.

Rich's family had two boats. One was a large wooden boat with a 75 horsepower outboard engine. The other was a new fiberglass runabout with a fifty horsepower outboard engine, and it was the one we liked to use. It was great for water skiing and fishing. The newer boat only had seats for four. Sometimes more people would show up and we would take the large wooden boat, but it was older and not very attractive.

Lake Hopatcong is one of New Jersey's largest lakes. It is about an hour north of Somerville, in a very nice part of New Jersey. There is a state Park there and, in those days, there was an amusement park on the lake. You could reach the park by boat and it had rides, games, and a roller coaster. Most Friday nights, we would load up the beer in a cooler, jump in the fiberglass boat, and head to the amusement park. Of course, we drank a bit on the way.

We always had a great time at the lake. We would go to the amuse-ment park, Bertram's Island, and if there were no girls there, we would ride around the lake looking for parties. One time we found a party and started singing our high school alma mater obnoxiously loud. Eventually, the people at the party invited us in. It happened to be a party of teachers, and they offered us beer. We said no thanks, we brought our own. Everyone laughed as we lifted the cooler out of the boat.

We partied for some time before heading back to Rich's place. The next morning we drove around the lake, looking for the place where the party was. When we found it, someone had backed a boat into the boathouse, and it had sunk. We stopped by and offered to help with the boat. While we were there, we met the teacher who hosted the party. Her name was Mickey, and she wasn't much older than we were. The house was her parents' summer home. She invited us to stop by whenever we wanted. She was a knockout, and we stopped by every once in a while to see her.

My junior year, Rich invited me to spend the summer at the lake house. I thought it would be great fun to water ski, fish, and chase girls, so I took him up on his invitation. That was the first summer I didn't play baseball or basketball.

I think that Rich's parents liked me. They were an Italian couple, and man, could Mrs. Panone cook. Mr. Panone owned a furniture store in Bound Brook, and the family seemed pretty well off. Rich had an older brother and a much younger sister. His brother Bob was married and had a couple of young daughters. He had married a girl whose brother was a friend of mine. They all used to show up on the weekends, and I didn't mind at all, because Linda would put on her bikini and tan herself down by the water. She certainly was a beautiful sight. Besides, Mrs. Panone would do a lot of good cooking for us.

During the week, Rich and I would ride around the lake looking for girls, because you needed at least three people to water ski. We did a lot of water skiing. I also did a lot of fishing. Living on a lake was still a dream of mine.

There was a place on the lake that you could go by boat and pick up a sandwich or soda. We stopped there quite often, because there was a girl working there that we enjoyed seeing. Her parents owned the place, and the bar that was upstairs. Her name was Diane James, and Rich and I both liked her. After the summer ended, I did get to date her, but the long trip to the lake got old pretty quickly.

Diane would travel to Somerville every once in awhile. Once, when Mark and I were passing through Lake Hopatcong, we stopped by Diane's house to see if she was home. Well, she was home, but she also had some guy over. So we politely said our hellos and goodbyes.

Shortly after that, she showed up at my house one day when I had a guest over. I guess we understood each other, and that was the last time I saw her. When I was much older, I moved to the lake, not far from Diane's house. I asked a friend about her, and was told that she'd married a doctor and they had a couple of kids. I'm sure that her parents were happy. I always felt that her parents did not approve of me.

◆　　　◆　　　◆

Rich and I met a lot of girls at the lake, and I thought everything was going along pretty well. Then, one day Rich got upset with me, saying I got to choose first whenever we met girls. I told him that I didn't care, and he could have the cutest girls. I just didn't care.

Two of the girls got pretty friendly and joined us wherever we went. We would take them on the boat at night to an isolated beach. We would make out, and I think they were pretty serious about us, but Rich and I would still go looking for other girls. At some point, they either got the hint or they went home, because we didn't see them again.

Many a Friday night during our lake parties, Rich would get really weird. He would crawl under a car and bark like a dog. All of us would think something was wrong, but he always straightened out by morning. We just assumed the beer had something to do with his behavior. Some years ago, I was told that Rich had passed away from some strange cancer.

I will never forget that summer spent fishing and chasing girls. What else could you ask for?

◆　　　◆　　　◆

As I mentioned, Chip went back to college. He attended Northwestern College, a small school in Iowa. I think he coached some baseball and majored in physical education. The best thing that happened to him was that he met a nice girl from Iowa, and Cathy became my sister-in-law. They got married in Florida and have two beautiful children, Shay and Adam.

Shay and Adam take after their father and are both pretty athletic. Shay played volleyball in high school and accepted a scholarship to play at Rider College in New Jersey. She was named captain of the team in her first year. She finished her education at Fort Lewis College in Durango, Colorado.

Adam, all six feet and nine inches of him, played soccer and basketball in high school. I watched him play several times, and I could tell he was better than his coach realized. He went to Fort Lewis College, where he still holds a record for percentage of shots taken and made. He finished his accounting degree at the University of Colorado at Colorado Springs.

When I graduated from high school, my mother moved to Florida to help my grandfather, who had built a house there. He had lived alone ever since my grandmother died. But life is funny sometimes, and before my mother actually got to Florida, my grandfather had hooked up with some lady that he'd known a long time ago. They got married and moved to another part of Florida. So my mother was by herself in the Florida house.

During the summer after graduation, I stayed in Somerville with my Aunt Margie and Uncle Phil and worked for the town. I picked up garbage and lined baseball fields. At two bucks an hour, for forty hours a week, I was saving more money than I ever had.

One night in December, when I was a senior in high school, Mark, Stan Jackowski and I were just riding around. Someone said, "Let's go to Barbara Dellavalle's house." She was a good-looking cheerleader who was a year behind us. So we all said, "Sure, let's go." When we got there, she had a friend over. Now, I told you to remember the name Jill Neumann, the girl I took to the freshman dance. We were all just kidding around, talking and cutting up. Well, before I knew what was going on, Mark and Stan were performing a fake wedding. Jill and I were the bride and groom. It was a lot of fun and quite funny.

In the three years since our first date, Jill and I had always been friendly, saying hi to each other at school. But this night seemed special, somehow. Jill and I became a couple, and I gave her my class ring. We stayed together all through the school year and the summer. Her parents owned a house at the Jersey Shore, and after work on Friday nights I would drive to the shore and spend the weekend there. Her parents didn't seem to mind me being around. I got along pretty well with her mom, but her father didn't bother with me much.

After the summer, we were getting ready to head to college, and we both were going to West Virginia. I was attending a Baptist college in Salem, West Virginia. Jill was attending a small college about forty miles away in Elkins.

I had to leave for school early in August, but Jill did not have to report to college until sometime in September. My Uncle Phil and Aunt Margie drove me to West Virginia to start my college career.

I had noticed a slight, strange feeling in my back before I left for school. It felt like a pulled muscle, and I figured it would just go away. I could have hurt myself anytime. During one football game, I was tackled out of bounds, and an opposing player speared me with his helmet right on the butt. It really hurt, but I continued to play. That was in the fall of my senior year, and after that I played a whole season of basketball and baseball. Still, if this was a football injury, it should have shown up much earlier. The only other discomfort I remember feeling was while I worked for the city, climbing in and out of a large dump truck. The pain got a little worse every day.

Now that I was at college, my back really started to bother me. I had to warm up a long time before I could do anything.

My roommates at school were nice. Each room had three guys in it, and one of my roommates was a big fellow. He decided that he was going to play college football, even though he hadn't played in high school. I figured it would take him a week to quit. He only lasted two days. My other roommate was older, on the small size, and acted sort of gay. He had transferred from a culinary school. But since he was older, he could have his car at school, which came in handy, and on several occasions we made the forty mile trip to see Jill.

The guys living across the hall were more to my liking. Two of the guys were from Jersey, and the third guy was from upstate New York. I got along better with them than I did with my roommates.

I kept a big picture of Jill on my desk. The guys would always ask me what Jill and I did sexually, which I thought was pretty rude. I felt you shouldn't disrespect your girl. Whether we were doing anything or not, it was certainly none of their business.

I had planned to play college basketball and baseball, but not football. I was six feet one inch, and weighed about 165 pounds, which was okay for high school, but not heavy enough for college football. One of the high school basketball players from a neighboring town, who was also on the All-County team, was going to play at this college. He was tall, but not such a great player. He had to go to school during the summer, and when he didn't return, I was hoping to pick up his scholarship.

By the time basketball season was about to start, my back was really uncomfortable. And then there was lack of money. My big savings account was gone in about three weeks. I called my mother, who was in Florida, to see what I should do. She said she would send me money to fly to Florida, and I agreed. The day I was to leave school, I received checks from my father, my uncle, and my mother. I left anyway. Actually the day, I left was the first day of basketball tryouts. I called Jill and told her I was leaving school to go to Florida.

When I got to Florida, I thought I'd better get my back pain checked out. The town my mother lived in was a very small gulf-side town with one doctor. I went to see him, and he said that there was nothing he could do about my back. That doctor was an idiot. My back was really bothering me, and at the very least he should have referred me to another doctor who could help me. I found out later that the same doctor was my grandmother's physician, and she died shortly after seeing him. I don't know whether or not he had anything to do with her death, but I guess I can say that now because I am sure that he is no longer alive.

So there I was in Florida not doing much of anything but fishing. I fished in the morning, and I fished at night. We lived not far from Lemon Bay, and it was like lake fishing, but with much bigger fish. I wasn't really looking for any type of work, just hanging out and fishing. My mother was working for a small insurance company in town.

My back was getting worse, and sometimes my brother would have to carry me to the pier where we fished. My brother lived with his wife in the next town to the north, in the middle of an orange grove. We saw each other quite often.

I met some pretty interesting old-timers on the pier. We would talk for hours about life and fishing. I would hope they taught me a lot about both. Sometimes I would clean the fish and cook them. It was a good way to supplement the grocery bill.

One of the old-timers had throat cancer. His operation had left just the hole where he could breath, and if he covered it, he could talk. I smoked at the time, and he would ask me for a drag. He would put the cigarette in the hole and take his drag, saying, "Don't tell my wife." I figured he had gone through a lot, and he was old. It made him happy, so I would always give him a drag.

I had spent several weeks in Florida. One afternoon, as I was getting ready to go fishing, the phone rang. My mother answered the phone and said, "I think it's Jill." I thought to myself, Isn't it nice that she's calling to see how I am? When I answered the phone, Jill wasn't her jovial self. She was still at school in West Virginia, but said she had something important to tell me. I braced myself for the worst, and asked her what was wrong. She told me we were going to be parents. I certainly wasn't expecting that, but we had always talked about marriage, so it just would be sooner than we thought. We decided that she would come to Florida and we would get married. But first she had to tell her parents.

Jill's family lived pretty well. Her father was an airline pilot, and her mother was a homemaker with three children. Jill was their middle child, with an older sister and a much younger brother. Her brother, Scott, was only about five years old.

I wasn't there when she told them, and I was glad of it. Of course, her parents were not thrilled. I really couldn't blame them. I mean, here's their daughter, tall, slender, and beautiful, and smart as a whip. She was going to school to become a nurse, had been voted most popular in our senior class, and was the head majorette. And now she was going to marry a college dropout with no job and a back injury. I would have been upset, too.

CHAPTER 5
Jill and Kane

Jill arrived in Florida, and we began making plans for the wedding. We visited the local Methodist church to see if we could be married there. At first, the minister said we were too young and he wouldn't perform our ceremony. But once we explained that we were expecting, he agreed. Then the minister gave me a long lecture on the sexual needs of a woman, which I thought was quite odd. I'm sure that on occasion Jill wished I had listened more carefully.

Jill's parents and her older sister, Candace, came to Florida for the wedding. One day, while we were sitting on the Englewood beach, beside the beautiful Gulf of Mexico, Jill's father offered me some money to just leave. Of course, I didn't accept.

In the small Methodist church, with just the eight of us, Jill and I were married. Candace was her maid of honor, and Chip was my best man. After the wedding, Mr. and Mrs. Neumann treated us all to a nice dinner. The next day Jill's folks left, and we started our life together. We were living with my mother. I had no job, and my back wasn't getting any better. I was still doing a lot of fishing and cooking what I caught.

Jill and my mother didn't get along too well. I don't know, or don't remember, how we got the money, but we decided to go back to New Jersey. In order to get our life on track, I had to get my back fixed. We flew back to New Jersey, and moved in with Jill's parents in Somerville.

The first or second day we were back in New Jersey, I went to see a neurosurgeon. He told me to go back home and lay on a board for two weeks without moving, and then let him know how I felt. I did what he asked, but in two weeks I felt the same, or maybe a little worse. I went back to the doctor. He said we should run some tests, and I agreed. But he seemed more concerned about being paid than about my health. Could the fact that I had no job, no money, no insurance, and no other way to pay him have been the cause? I promised him he would get paid, and we scheduled the tests. I didn't know how I was going to pay for them, but I knew we had to do something with my back.

The doctor admitted me to the local hospital for testing. They inserted dye into my back, and then elevated me to watch the dye flow down my spine. As we watched on a TV screen, the dye hit a certain spot and seemed to spread out all over the place. When this happened, the doctor wrote a bunch of stuff on my back. The procedure to inject the dye into my back hadn't been pleasant, and I was in a lot of pain. The doctor seemed to think I was some kind of wimp, but let me tell you, it really hurt.

After the test, the doctor told me I had a disk problem and he would have to operate the following day. He gave me a fifty-fifty chance that the operation would be successful. At that point, I felt those were pretty good odds. Besides, what did I have to lose? I could barely walk.

The next day I went in for the operation. At first, an orderly came into the room and said he had to give me an enema. I wasn't real sure what that was, but I soon found out. He not only gave me one, but he had to do a second. I think he really enjoyed it. It was such a pleasant experience. Then they took me into surgery. I don't know how long I was in the operating room or the recovery room. They actually removed the damaged disk, but didn't fuse the vertebrae with a piece of bone from my hip like they normally did. The doctor told me that I was young enough that the bones would fuse in time by themselves.

When I came out of the recovery room, Jill was waiting. My brother and mother were also there. They had moved back from Florida and were living in the same apartment complex where Chip and I had grown up. I was still under the influence of the drugs, and I was quite happy and feeling no pain. They transferred me to a room, and I slept for a long time.

A big, fat nurse woke me up and said that I would have to void. I said, "What?" She told that I would have to urinate. I said, "I haven't had any water, and I don't have to go."

She said, "If you don't go, we'll have to stick a tube up your penis." Then she left the room.

The guy in the neighboring bed spoke up, saying, "I had that done yesterday, and it's not pleasant." Quick thinker that I am, I asked him to pee in the urinal for me. He said he shouldn't do that because he had diabetes. I asked him if he would help me try to go. He agreed, and I told him to get a warm glass of water to pour on my penis as I tried to use the urinal.

We were doing that when the nurse came in and yelled, "What are you guys doing?" To this day, I don't know if I went, but there was something in the urinal, and the nurse just looked at it and flushed whatever it was.

Later that night, the nurse came in and said that I would have to get up and walk. I wasn't too sure about that plan, but I got up and I walked. I had absolutely no pain, and felt as though I could have run if they'd asked. I only spent three or four days in the hospital.

After I'd been home a day or two, some friends came over, and we went out and played basketball. I guess that wasn't real smart, since I still had the stitches in my back, but I felt fine. It was about time. Things were looking up for a change.

I was really getting along well with Jill's mother, but her father was a different story. Basically, I think he just didn't like me, and he thought I was an immature little wiseass. Which, in retrospect, I guess I was.

One day I was sitting in the kitchen drinking a soda. Mr. Neumann came in and asked me, "How ambitious do you feel?"

Being eighteen years old, I said, "Not very." Mr. Neumann stomped off as though he was really mad. A little later, Mrs. Neumann told me that he only wanted me to wash the car, which I did immediately. If he had asked, I would have done it gladly. I guess he thought I was a mind reader.

My back was better, and it was time to find a job. I thought finding a job in my hometown would be a snap. I knew a lot of people, and a lot of people knew me because of sports. There I was, thinking again. I couldn't even find a job shoveling poop. In desperation, I went to an employment agency and paid to get a job. It never ends, does it?

In a week or so, I had a job as a clerk at the Formica Corporation warehouse. Jill was getting pretty big. Her paternal aunt was an obstetrical nurse. She helped us get discounts on all the doctor visits and the delivery. The only catch was that we had to have the baby at the hospital where she worked. Kennedy hospital was located in Edison, New Jersey. It was a few miles away, but the price was right.

It was March, 1968, when I got a call at work from Jill. The baby was coming. I remember it like it was yesterday. I drove home to take Jill to the hospital, but Mrs. Neumann wanted to drive. I thought that was my job, so she agreed to follow us. At the hospital, they said I was too young to go into the delivery room. I thought that was pretty ridiculous, since I'd been old enough to make the baby. As usual, I was passive, and I sat and waited. I don't remember much about the wait, just hearing a few screams and being told I had a son.

Jill and I were blessed, and he was healthy. We had long discussions about what to name him. We finally chose Kane. It was Jill's mother's maiden name, and I thought the name was manly. The Kane name was well known in the neighboring township of Hillsborough. Jill's grandfather had been a judge there at one time. He also ran the school buses for the whole Township. Besides being a cool name, I felt Kane was also a tribute to Jill's grandparents and mother.

Kane was a great kid, and I just knew he would be a great athlete. I truly thought that he had good athletic skills, and as time went by, he showed me exactly that. When he was four, I would throw baseballs to him. The kid could really hit the ball.

Kane's mother didn't think much of sports. She would say to me, "What good are all those sports doing for you now?" I had to agree that it might have been better if I had learned some type of trade, but I felt that athletics had taught me a lot about life. For instance, I learned my determination to succeed from playing sports. I guess Jill just couldn't see the value of sports. So Kane was never really given a chance. Still, Jill did a great job with him. He became a great person, and a successful adult.

◆   ◆   ◆

Things were not going well at Jill's parents' house. Her father and I were just not getting along. One day, he had given me money to rent a wet/dry vacuum. I thought I knew where the rental store was, but I couldn't find it. So I came home, put the money on the fireplace mantle, and was going to go out again. As I was leaving, he was headed up the stairs. He asked me how I did, and I told him. He started yelling that I was incompetent and immature. Jill's mother had to step in and stop us, because I called Mr. Neumann out. I would have fought him. We did not speak to or see each other for four years. When Jill took Kane to see her parents, I didn't go.

Jill and I agreed it was time to get our own apartment. After working several months, we had saved some money. Jill's parents also said they would give her one thousand dollars to help set up an apartment. But Jill had to promise not to use the money to pay off my operation. My mother actually stepped in and said she would make monthly payments to the doctor. So Jill, Kane, and I moved into the apartment complex where I had grown up. Actually, we weren't far from my Uncle Phil, my mother, and my brother.

We now had a one-bedroom apartment on a tree-lined street. Jill's parents were pretty generous. Besides the thousand dollars, they gave us their 1960 Pontiac Bonneville. So there we were, on our own. I went to work, and Jill stayed at home and took care of the baby. That was the way I thought it should be.

After a couple of job changes, I found myself working at Somerset Trust Company. Finally, being a Somerville athlete really helped. The president of the bank knew me because of sports. I don't think he realized that I'd dated his daughter briefly in high school. She was a year older, and gorgeous. One afternoon we were in their rec room, smooching a little. One of her older brothers came in and caught us. He threw me out of the house, slamming the door and yelling, "Don't you ever come back." That was the last time I saw her socially.

I got along fine with the president, who once taught me a very important lesson. I've rarely followed it, but have never forgotten it. He said, "You don't shit where you eat, and you don't eat where you shit."

◆   ◆   ◆

About this time, Jill and I moved to an apartment attached to a house. The owner lived in the main house. She was a single mother with three kids. The house was located in Bridgewater Township. It was a little more country than the apartments, so we had a large front yard, and a large backyard bordering a small wooded area. We enjoyed living there and got along well with the owner.

◆   ◆   ◆

I had started working at a bank as a credit trainee, which was a grooming position for becoming a bank officer. I was the youngest of three trainees. The two older trainees would spend a week in each department, but since I was less experienced, I spent a month in each department. That was okay with me, because it was a great opportunity to learn.

After about six months, the bank discontinued the training program and placed the three of us in different jobs. Because I was the youngest, they transferred me to the teller line. I wasn't real happy there, but I stuck it out. I worked at the Finderne branch, which was one of the busiest branches in the bank. Before long, I was promoted to head teller.

After a year or so, I got a call from Tom Sullivan, vice president and head of the mortgage department. He invited me to lunch and offered me a job in the mortgage department. The job meant a bigger paycheck, and Tom was a real nice guy. When he told me that people who had previously held the position he was offering me were now officers of the bank, I took him up on his offer.

Jill's grandfather had decided to sell a house he owned in Hillsborough Township, so we went to see it. Jill just fell in love with it, and I liked it, too. It sat on almost an acre of land out in the country. The house was a large Cape Cod, with two roomy bedrooms upstairs and two more bedrooms downstairs. There was an unfinished full basement and a little sunroom off the west side of the house. I had great plans to make that room into a bar, but the rest of the house needed a little work first.

Jill asked her parents to help us buy the house. They gave her the money that had been in her college fund. With that for a down payment, and a mortgage from my bank, we bought our first house.

My father helped me fix it up. We made that sunroom into one cool place of entertainment and spirits. We put in blue paneling, red curtains, and, of course, a bar I bought at Sears. We also got a riding lawn mower so I could cut the grass on our little acre.

Kane started school, and Jill decided to go back to college. She attended the nursing program at the local community college, graduated, and became a licensed practical nurse. By this time we had two cars. I was still in the mortgage department, and Jill went to work at Somerville Hospital. With two salaries, we were doing pretty well. Actually, Jill was making a lot more than I was.

You would think that I had everything I could want, but that wasn't the case. I recently talked to Jill about this whole thing, and she basically said I didn't know how to be a father and husband because I had no real role model to follow. But what actually happened was that I became like my father, a drinker and womanizer. I guess I just didn't know what I wanted, and working at the bank with the parties and girls wasn't good for me.

Jill and I weren't getting along. One Sunday afternoon, we had a big fight. I don't remember what we were arguing about, but in the heat of the moment, Jill blurted, "Why don't you just leave?" She had a very sharp tongue and could make me feel I was just stupid. She used to act so superior, I often felt she and Kane would be better off without me.

Jill charged out, taking Kane to see her parents. I decided to leave, and packed my Volkswagen Bug with my clothes and fishing gear. I left everything else. Needless to say, moving out didn't endear me to Jill's father.

Jill's mother had taught her to cook, and when I left her, I weighed 220 pounds. After a few weeks of being out on my own, I dropped twenty-five pounds and was back to my fighting weight.

My mother had re-married George, which proved to be a good thing. Chip and I had our own families, and we hadn't paid much attention to Mom. She had started drinking quite a bit, and Poppa George came around just in time. They had moved to Plainfield, and said I could come and live with them. So, I moved back in with my mother.

Jill and I agreed that she and Kane would keep the house, and I would take all the other bills. I was concerned about what people would say, but Poppa George told me, "Don't worry about it. They will talk about you today, and somebody else tomorrow."

CHAPTER 6
Life after Jill

The commute from Plainfield to the bank was all of ten or fifteen miles, but it was really getting to me. Either that, or I just wanted to get out of my mother's house. A bunch of guys I knew were renting rooms from John Kitchen, a friend of my brother's. I asked him if I could rent a room. At first he was hesitant, but he finally gave in, and I moved into his house in Somerville. It was a nice house on the east end of High Street. There were a lot of medical and legal offices in the area. The house faced the county administration building across the street.

During the first couple of months, being on my own was really different. For one thing, I noticed that I became pretty horny. I went in search of someone to satisfy my needs, and the girls at the bars seemed to be looking for the same thing that I was. It didn't take long to remedy my situation, but the solution was always temporary.

There were four of us living in Kitchen's house. Bob Gardner and Ron Winkels were two of the guys. Ron, I knew from high school and football. Bob was my brother's age, and a real nice guy. Bob was about six feet three inches tall, enjoyed basketball, and had played in college. He went to a small school in Tennessee. Bob was prematurely balding, the same problem Chip was having.

Winks, as we all called him, was a redhead and a pretty tough guy. But his feet had an odor all their own. One day he fell asleep on the couch with his shoes off. The smell was so bad, we had to set the couch on the porch to air it out. We finally convinced Winks to go see a foot doctor. Reluctantly, he went to his appointment. As the doctor was examining Ron's feet, he kept looking around. When Ron asked him what he was looking for, the doctor said, "I'm looking for your wheelchair, because I know you didn't walk in here on these puppies."

The podiatrist found several types of fungi on Winks' feet. He cleared up his foot problems just in time, because Winks soon met Kathy and fell in love. I was there the first night they met. There was something special about the two of them. They married and had a beautiful daughter.

After a while, the friend who owned the house gave us notice that he was getting married, and we all had to move out. So Bob, Ron, and I got together and rented a house in Liberty Corners. The house had recently been renovated and had all new wood floors and a new bathroom. It was a two-story with four bedrooms upstairs, and was next door to the local deli. Now that was a bachelor pad.

I was seeing Kane as much as I could, but it probably wasn't enough. I went back one day to see if Jill wanted to reconcile. We talked for a while, but I felt as though she didn't want me back, so I never asked her about reconciliation.

Her father had always said, "Have an idea." Jill did, and I really couldn't blame her. Who knew what I was going to do? I didn't know myself. One time she asked me to baby-sit because she had to go somewhere. I figured it used to be my house, too, so I started snooping around and found men's clothes in the closet. They weren't mine. Jill did have an idea, and his name was Jeff. Again, I didn't blame her. Jeff lived at the Jersey Shore across the lagoon from Jill's parents. He and Jill had known each other for some time.

We got a divorce. I remember sitting in the courthouse, waiting for our attorneys. Jill and I were sitting on a bench together. I was lighting her cigarette when both attorneys came in. My attorney said, "Are you sure you want to get divorced? You guys look pretty happy." But we were only happy because we were getting a divorce.

Being in the banking business, borrowing came easily, and I borrowed to pay for the divorce. I was getting in pretty deep. In the divorce, I gave Jill and Kane the house. I didn't want Kane growing up in apartments like I had. And I'd taken over all our bills. Shortly after the divorce, Jill married Jeff. I really didn't mind. He was a good person, and I knew he would take good care of them.

Jill sold our house. She made some good money from the sale and told me she would put some of the profits in a college fund for Kane. I thought that was a great idea. Jill and Jeff bought a ranch house in Pluckemin. It was kind of country, and about five or six miles north of Somerville. Whenever I would pick Kane up or drop him off, Jeff would invite me in for a cocktail. It bothered me to sit at my own bar.

At one point, my debt was growing faster than my income, and I got a little behind in my child support payments. After I missed a few months, Jill came to me with an offer. If I let Jeff adopt Kane, I wouldn't have to pay the back child support.

Now, I have done a lot of bad things in my life, but what I agreed to then surpassed anything I had done up to that point, or anything I've done since. It really pains me deeply to talk about it. I agreed to let Jeff adopt Kane, but only with the stipulation that I got visitation rights.

I have recently talked to Kane and Jill both about this. I didn't try to justify why it happened. I just wanted to tell them how sorry I was that I let it happen. My reasoning at the time is irrelevant and doesn't change the end result. In retrospect, I'd rather have gone to jail for being a deadbeat dad. I certainly hope that Kane has forgiven me.

◆   ◆   ◆

In 1974, I was attending the banking school at Ohio State University. It was the National School of Real Estate Finance. This was shortly after my divorce from Jill, and I was interested in real estate finance. I had a six-foot six-inch roommate from New Jersey who had played basketball at Duke University. His senior year at Duke, he played in the NCAA Final Four. I don't recall if they went all the way, but he wore a watch that said he was there.

One particular morning, I woke up feeling as though I had a lot of blankets on me, but it was actually summer, and I only had a sheet on my legs. I thought it seemed odd, but I figured maybe it had something to do with my back operation in 1968. The sensation didn't affect my walking. As a matter of fact, that morning my roommate and I played basketball.

After finishing the college course, I returned to New Jersey and went to see the surgeon that operated on my back. He told me that the feeling was a side effect of the surgery and would go away. He also said that I'd eventually need another operation. After a few days, the numbness in my legs got better, but it stayed in my feet. I just figured that would eventually go away, too. It really didn't hinder my ability to walk or run, so I just ignored it.

Denial is a bad thing! The numbness stayed with me. I would occasionally get numbness in my fingers, too, but that was sporadic and always went away. It wasn't anything that I couldn't handle. I just reminded myself that the surgeon said it would go away.

◆　　　◆　　　◆

Because of sports, I've been very fortunate to meet and play against some pretty famous people. During my senior year in high school, we played basketball at South River. I remember seeing lots of signs and banners about Joe Somebody. Only later did I figure out who was actually on that team. I think I may have guarded him during the game. I do remember that we won.

Now, every time he comes on TV, I tell the boys that I played basketball against that guy. Can you guess who this famous person is? After high school, where he was an all-state quarterback, he went to Notre Dame University and played four years there. He was most remembered for breaking his leg when Lawrence Taylor tackled him on national television. He also quarterbacked the Washington Redskins to a Super Bowl victory. He now does football announcing on ESPN. That's right, Joe Theismann.

Two months after my back operation, in 1968, Jill's best friend, Diane, told me that her father wanted to talk to me. He asked me if I wanted to play basketball for the dairy where he worked. It was only one game, with a party afterward at the owner's home. Of course I said yes.

When I got there, I was introduced to the other players, and one name really stuck out from the rest. Ralph Terry, the great Yankee pitcher, had only been retired for a year, and being a Yankee fan, I was well aware of who he was. I don't remember anything about the game, but I remember going to the owner's home, which was more of a mansion than a house. I remember sitting and talking to Mr. Terry at the party. He'd married the daughter of the owner of the dairy. We talked baseball, and I mentioned that my brother was playing for the Houston organization. I got Mr. Terry's autograph for my son, and have since learned that Kane's mother still has it. One other thing that really impressed me about that evening was how gorgeous Mrs. Terry was.

During my junior and senior years playing basketball, there was a fellow named Billy Garland on the team. He was a year behind me and was a great basketball player. There were a lot of things that Billy had that all us white boys wanted. Even though he was only six feet two inches tall, he could dunk the ball with two hands. He also had a fade-away jump shot that could not be blocked, and he was the first Somerville High basketball player to score 1000 points or more. After graduation, he attended the local junior college, and for a few games he was the leading scorer in the nation. I lost track of him over the years, but during a visit with a friend of mine from Somerville, I learned that Billy had a son named Tupac Shakur.

I was very fortunate to be asked to play on certain teams quite often after high school graduation, thanks to my friend and basketball mentor, Leon Mintschenko. He had moved to Somerville from Australia when he was twelve years old, and had never picked up a basketball until then. He was two years ahead of me in high school, and also played football and baseball, but not as well as he did basketball. He was only five feet eleven inches, but he could really play basketball. His senior year he was All-State, and I was a sophomore playing JV. Toward the end of the season, Leon sprained his ankle pretty badly. Since Leon was injured, the coach asked me if I wanted to dress for the varsity games, which, of course, was the dream of any underclass basketball player. So I got to dress for two games, and even played in one of them.

After graduation, Leon went to the University of Rhode Island, where he played for four years. He also married a cheerleader and friend of mine, Patty, from Somerville. She and Leon had three children. Unfortunately, Leon suffered a heart attack a couple of years ago and passed away. I don't think I go a day without thinking about him. Leon used to ask me to play on teams that played against professional players of other sports besides basketball. One time we played against the 1969 New York Mets team and players like Ron Swoboda, Bud Harrelson, and Ed Cranepool. We actually won that game, and the Mets were not happy. After all, a lot of people had come and paid to see them. Too bad!

Leon also asked me to play with the high school teachers against the New York Giants football team. Running back Ron Johnson, defensive back Spider Lockhart, and center Bob Highland played. We lost that one. And later, with the high school teachers' team, we played the Arkansas Lassies, a professional women's basketball team. They cheated and played routines like the Harlem Globe Trotters, like trying to pull your shorts down as you shot free throws. Needless to say, we lost that game, too.

Back in 1976, when I first moved to Colorado, my brother helped me get on a basketball team in town. There was a real ball hog named Rich "Goose" Gossage who played on that team. At that time he was still with the Chicago White Sox, but soon after that he signed with the New York Yankees. He was a great relief pitcher and will be in the Hall of Fame soon. He still lives here in Colorado Springs, and does a lot for the kids in town.

◆　　　◆　　　◆

Now, back to beautiful downtown Liberty Corners, which was a little place. It did have a post office, a barbershop, and one small market. Liberty Corners was famous for the birth of quintuplets, and it wasn't far from the PGA headquarters, Jackie O's home, and Mike Tyson's first house.

Bob, Winks, and I were still playing sports. We played touch football, industrial league basketball, and softball. I really enjoyed the softball. It's much faster than hardball and is a lot of fun. The three of us used to hang out at a local tavern called The Old York Inn, just west of the town of Raritan, and not far from John Basalone's statue.

Bob didn't drink often, but Winks and I did. Bob was a little older than us and watched over us to make sure we didn't do anything too stupid.

The Old York Inn, run by the three Maxwell brothers, was a great place to hang out. It was a very sports-oriented place, and both Winks and I had the pleasure of bartending there on occasion. The money really came in handy then, and the experience came in handy later. It was a great place to meet friends and have a beer or two. Draft beer cost a quarter a glass when I first started hanging out there. Plus, they served a great pizza pie. The Old York Inn had a softball team, and the three of us played on it. We never partied before the games, but we sure partied after them. The three of us shared some good times, and we still try to keep in touch.

Bob, Winks, and I used to go on road trips during three-day weekends. One time, over a long weekend, we headed to Maine in Bob's International Scout. We found a place on the Maine coast called Christmas Cove. It was beautiful there, and the motel and restaurant were right on the water.

Before we got there, we stopped in a small town, picked up a bottle of wine and some cheese, and ate in a church parking lot. When we got to the motel, Winks got violently ill. So, Bob and I left him there, went to the restaurant, and had a great lobster dinner. The three of us traveled around Maine, did some trout fishing, and actually caught a few. We spent some time at Rangley Lake and did some more fishing. It was a great trip.

One time during January, Bob and I decided to go to Disney World. Our other passenger was Bob's dog, Tara, a weimaraner. It was a very cold morning when we hopped into my VW bug and headed south. We were in winter coats. By the time we hit South Carolina, we had stripped down to tee shirts. In Florida, we stopped in Titusville, where a girl Bob knew lived. He called her, and they visited for a while before we headed to Disney World, which was brand new. We had good time there, too.

After Disney World, we headed to Tampa, where we visited Busch Gardens. Tara wasn't allowed to go into the park, so Bob put her in a kennel. I guess she didn't like that, so she pooped and then rolled in it. She was a smelly mess, and Bob had to use a hose to clean her off before we could let her back in the car.

The VW was a little cramped, especially with Tara in the back seat. We decided to head south to see where I used to live with my mother and Jill. We spent some time there and, of course, did some fishing before heading back to New Jersey.

During the spring of 1975, Bob and I took two weeks of vacation and headed to Colorado. We decided to drive Bob's 1971 Porsche 911 Targa. The car was yellow with a black Targa top, and it was sweet.

We were going to my brother's place in Colorado Springs. The trip west was beautiful, and it only took us two days to get to Rocky Mountain National Park. We stayed there just a short time, and then headed south toward Colorado Springs.

We visited with my brother and made day trips to go fishing in the mountains. One day we were at Eleven Mile Reservoir. The air is pretty thin up there, and the Porsche just would not run. We had a heck of a time getting back to the Springs. But we did get some fishing done. One morning in Eleven Mile Canyon, Bob and I caught and released over ninety trout. We didn't see another fisherman all day. Overall, it was a good trip.

◆　　　　◆　　　　◆

At the time of my separation and divorce from Jill, I was still working at the bank. Of course, I was interested in the ladies and had dated several employees. Then I met a girl named Karen through a mutual friend. Karen was a cute little thing with curly brown hair, who lived with her folks in Manville. She had just separated from her husband, Bill, who I'd known in high school. I remember once during football practice in my sophomore year, Bill was holding a blocking pad, and somebody hit him hard enough to break his arm. We were showering after practice, and he came back from the hospital, overjoyed that he wouldn't have to practice anymore. That didn't sit well with me. Consequently, I always thought Bill was a little weird. Karen and I saw each other several times while they were separated. One night, I was eating dinner at the bar in The Old York Inn. I always sat with my back to the wall, since I was taught never to sit with my back to the door. If you're from New Jersey, you'll understand. Out of the corner of my eye, I saw Bill walk in. He wasn't a regular at The Old York Inn. I knew something was going to happen.

Bill was not very tall, sort of stocky, and looked more than a little upset. There were plenty of stools available, but he sat down right next to me. Someone had told him that I was seeing his estranged wife. I was a little nervous, but he was shaking. After sitting down, he asked me if I had seen Karen lately. I told him that I had not, which was true. He didn't say another word, but he kept playing with my dinner knife on the bar, looking as though he wanted to hurt me. I suggested that he not do anything stupid, and with that, he put the knife down, got up, and left. I never saw him again, but after that I became very cautious about dating married ladies.

I did have a serious relationship for a couple of years with a girl named Linda who worked at the bank. Linda was from Princeton, New Jersey, and had attended high school there. She told me that during her high school years she was a little overweight, but by the time I met her she was cute and nicely built. She had a little butt, and my nickname for her was LB.

I asked her to marry me. She was pretty smart and said no several times. I had met her parents and gotten the feeling that they didn't like me. She had two brothers, one older and one younger. Her father was a psychiatrist, and the family wasn't real pleased that I had been married. They were Catholic folks, and they frowned upon that for their daughter.

Linda actually did say yes to one of my proposals, but by that time I knew the relationship wasn't going to work out, and I stopped seeing her. I heard that she married an attorney and had a couple of daughters. I am sure that made her family happy. When I saw them a few years later at a social event, Linda and her husband did not talk to me. They sure gave me dirty looks, though, and I don't know what they were upset about. After all, if it hadn't been for me, they wouldn't be together.

◆   ◆   ◆

I was still working at the bank and moving up the corporate ladder. Tom Sullivan had been promoted, and the bank was looking for his replacement as head of the mortgage department. I really thought that I should be promoted.

I didn't get the job, and I was a little upset about it. They promoted an older guy who had been with the bank for many years. I tried, but I could not work with him. He was more interested in making little characters out of nuts than in running the department, and he would do that all day long at his desk. I decided I had wasted nearly five years in the department, so I made a few phone calls to let the higher ups know that I wanted out.

I learned many years later that the powers-to-be felt I was completely out of control because of my social behavior after work. I didn't think I was out of control just because I drank a little and was seeing two girls from the bank at the same time, but, as far as they were concerned, I was.

So, I moved into operations as an assistant manager of a branch office at the shopping center in Bridgewater Township. I was still attracted to a pretty face, and Anna, a teller at the branch office, caught my eye. Her teller station was in front of my desk. All day long, I would sit there looking at Anna and her butt. She was blonde and well-built. A customer used to call her the Bionic Woman, because she looked like Lindsey Wagner the star of that TV show. But we both worked for the bank, and dating a fellow employee was frowned upon.

I thought Anna would be a great person for Bob to date, and I set up a meeting for them. Now, Bob was a little older and much more mature. He suffered from a lack of hair follicles. After they met, Anna told me that he was too old for her, so I asked her out. She said yes, and we dated for some time.

Around this time, Bob bought a house south of Bound Brook. It was a three-bedroom ranch, so Winks and I rented rooms from him. I was getting real tired of the single life and bachelorhood. I truly thought that Anna would be a good one to settle down with. She had five siblings: two older brothers, a younger brother, and two younger sisters. We spent a lot of time at her parents' home.

Her parents were from Poland. They could speak English, but whenever I was around, they spoke Polish. Her father used to call me the playboy with the little red sports car, because at the time I was driving a red Porsche 914. I didn't think I deserved either the name or their obvious opinion of me. They would talk about me in Polish while

I was sitting there. After a while, I started to understand what they were saying.

To make a long story short, I proposed, and she said yes. We went to her folks to plan the wedding. Her father said, "You plan everything, and I will pay for it." After we had all the plans made, her father came to us and said he did not like what we were serving at the reception. We didn't want to change the meal. He said, "If that's the case, I will not pay for it." We decided to pay for things ourselves, and the plans went ahead. Even though her folks didn't like me, we still got married in the little Methodist Church in Somerville on April 3, 1976.

The reception was held at the Jolly Ox Restaurant in Hillsborough. The owner, a friend of mine, had worked at the bank. He gave us a real good deal on the reception. It was quite an affair. All our friends were invited, and we sure had a good time, especially with the open bar.

We honeymooned in Florida. We went to Disney World and Lemon Bay and fished for a few days. But somehow the relationship didn't seem to start off right.

By this time I had become an officer of the bank, assistant treasurer, and managed a small branch in Martinsville. Anna and I had rented an apartment in an old house in Bound Brook. We lived on the bottom floor, and the second floor had three apartments, occupied by an old lady and two young guys. After I had moved to the apartment a couple months before the wedding, some very strange things had gone in the old house. First of all, one night just as I was falling asleep, I saw a ghost at the foot of the bed. Now, I swear this is absolutely true, and that is no bull poop. I had not been drinking, and I was lying in bed going to sleep. Don't laugh. I could tell it was a lady's form, standing there, looking at me. There were little lights all around her. I was scared and didn't know what to think. Then the apparition just turned and walked out of the room. After that, I started sleeping with a Bible under my pillow, along with my BB gun.

As time went by, Anna and I would find things missing, like canned goods. One day I went to the freezer to get a package of chicken breast fillets I had put there three days earlier. As I touched the package, I realized it wasn't frozen. All of the other items I'd purchased that day were frozen. At first we thought it was the guys upstairs or even the old lady. But our liquor supply was not touched, which eliminated the young guys.

We started to stick match heads at the top of one of the two doors going into the apartment. We figured if we found a match head on the floor when we got home, someone had been in the apartment. We did it every day for two weeks, and there was absolutely no sign of entry. Very strange!

◆   ◆   ◆

The numbness in my feet and hands had stayed the same. It wasn't any worse, and didn't bother me at all. I was still in denial.

I was now playing softball for a new team, sponsored by a fancy restaurant in Somerville called La Brochette. The owner's son, Nick Bissell, Jr., was a local attorney. He managed the team and played, too. He wasn't that athletic, but he knew how to treat his teammates. They were mostly lawyers and county probation workers. Bob Gardner, a probation officer, had asked me to play with them. We weren't that good, but we had a lot of fun. Nick supplied the team with four sets of uniforms. His secretary called each of us on game day to let us know which uniform to wear.

A few years ago, I was watching the news and heard something about Somerville, New Jersey, so I listened up. I really don't know the complete story, but I'll tell you what I found out.

Nick had become the District Attorney for the county. I guess he was a pretty tough D.A. and made a lot of enemies. Then he and a friend of his opened a gas station in town. Whatever happened with the money and the gas station, Nick was placed under house arrest. He had one of those ankle monitors on so they'd know if he went anywhere. Apparently convinced he was going to jail, Nick cut the monitor off, got into his car, and headed west. He made it to Las Vegas before they caught up with him. As the story goes, Nick had some fun, then when the authorities knocked on his door, he told them he would not be taken alive. As the police entered, they heard a gunshot and found Nick dead. Whenever I go back to Somerville and mention Nick's name, people refuse to talk about him.

◆   ◆   ◆

Chip and my Uncle Bill had moved to Colorado. Uncle Bill moved because Johns Manville offered him and his wife both jobs in the company's new facility in Denver. My brother, who was living in Iowa and driving a truck, decided to try out Colorado for a change of lifestyle.

Anna and I thought it might be nice to live in Colorado, too. I took a week off and flew to Colorado to check out job possibilities. I'd always thought that once you became a bank officer, finding another job would be a snap. After a week of interviews, I had nothing solid. But one bank did say it would be better if I were a Colorado resident.

When I got back home, Anna and I talked about moving to Colorado anyway. We decided to take a chance and move lock, stock, and barrel to Colorado. I resigned from the bank. We sold some of our things, packed up the rest, and headed out West in her 1974 Chevy Nova.

I remember being in Colorado and staying at Chip's house. I went to a lot of interviews, and we had some money from the things we had sold before we left. One of the things we sold was my Porsche, thinking it was better to have just one car to drive to Colorado.

After two weeks at my brother's, we decided to get our own apartment. We didn't move far, but we were on our own. Anna got a job pretty quickly as a teller in a bank. I drove her to work in the morning so that I had a car for job-hunting.

The apartment complex that we moved into had a clubhouse, a heated swimming pool, and a Jacuzzi. After taking Anna to work, I would go back to the clubhouse to read the classified ads and have coffee. There were several other guys there doing the same thing. And, of course, there were the cleaning girls and the managers who worked at the complex. After spending as much time as I did at the clubhouse, I got to know them all pretty well, but I wasn't fooling around or anything.

The most important thing I learned during that time in Colorado was that the mountains were beautiful, but you couldn't eat them. I went on countless interviews, with no results. One banker told me I should move to Grand Junction. He said they were looking for bankers because it was the fastest growing town in Colorado. Grand Junction was on the western slope, and I really didn't want to move there.

After I'd been looking for several months without finding a job, Anna and I were not getting along too well. She was stressed about being our sole support. Plus, she'd always been nervous about me cheating on her. Honest to God, I was not cheating on her. But another month went by without me getting a job, and things were getting pretty rough.

I finally did find a job in Pueblo, which is about forty miles south of the Springs. I was hired as an assistant manager at a finance company, but after two days of commuting to Pueblo, I realized I wouldn't be happy there. After being a banker for so long, I had a very difficult time calling people who were already late on their payments, encouraging them to come in and borrow more money. I realized the job wasn't going to work out.

Besides, there were a couple of ladies who had been with the company for quite a few years, and they seemed to think one of them should have been named assistant manager. I thought they were right. I resigned and went back to the clubhouse.

By this time, our financial situation was desperate. I talked to my mother. She and Poppa George had bought a ranch house on a large lot in a very upscale neighborhood in Plainfield. She told me if Anna and I would come back, we could stay with them. So we packed up the

Nova, and we headed back to New Jersey. Within two weeks, Anna and I had both gotten excellent jobs at different banks. Our jobs weren't in Somerville, but in Morristown, about 25 miles north.

I love my mother, but two families trying to live in one house usually doesn't work, and within a month we decided to get our own apartment again. We found a very nice one in Somerville, so we moved.

Once we were settled, we decided we needed a puppy. We went to the puppy farm and picked out our dog. She was a mix of German Shepherd and St. Bernard. She was real cute, but we knew that she was going to be big. We called her Farah, for Farah Fawcett, the actress. Eventually we started calling her Fa. It wasn't fair to the dog that we went off to work each day and left her alone, so we hired a neighbor kid to walk Fa before and after school. This dog was unbelievable. Once she ate the foam out of the couch cushions. I was amazed she could get the zippers open on the cushion covers.

Just before Christmas, Anna and I put up our first Christmas tree and decorations. When we got home from work the next day, to our shock, Farah had not only pulled the Christmas tree down, but she'd eaten all the balls and chewed the lights up.

One evening, we were out for a ride and, of course, Fa was with us. We drove past The Old York Inn, and by this time it was dark and past beer thirty. We decided to stop in for a beer or two. We promised Fa we wouldn't be long and told her she'd be okay in the car. Of course, we stayed longer than we should have. When we finally got to the car, Fa had eaten the interior of the passenger side door. She must have been really hungry, because she chewed right down to the metal. Anna's Chevy Nova was never the same.

It was amazing that the dog never got sick. She could eat anything. When we went out to dinner, we always brought home the baked potatoes, and Farah would feast on them.

I really enjoyed my new job at First Morris Bank. All the officers were about my age. The president was only thirty years old, and the staff all got along well. Anna's bank, Heritage North, was an older bank in downtown Morristown. We were only a few miles apart, and we could ride to work together.

Still, the bickering had never stopped after the Colorado episode. No matter what, she would tell me that I wasn't doing my job right and accuse me of getting too friendly with the tellers, who all happened to be young girls. It seemed the arguing was nonstop anytime we were together.

I don't think anger is one of the symptoms of multiple sclerosis. But I was real tired a lot of the time, and that might have contributed to my anger. Besides the tiredness, I still had some numbness in my hands and feet. These symptoms didn't bother me, though, and I just lived with them.

One day when I walked into the apartment, Anna was packing her bag. I asked her where was she going. She said, "I am just going away for a couple days." That was all she would say. I carried her bags to her car. I really didn't know where she was going, and I honestly didn't care. I realized I was hoping she didn't come back.

I had bought a 1972 Carmen Ghia convertible. One night during Anna's absence, I stopped on the way home from work and had a few drinks. I left the bar about one o'clock in the morning. The apartment was only a mile and a half away, down the same street. For some reason, when I got to the middle of Main Street, I decided I should go to the diner for breakfast instead of going home. My turn was not a great turn, but it wasn't a bad one, either.

As I was traveling down the street, I noticed a police car with its lights flashing. As the car pulled me over, I smiled to myself because I knew all the cops in town. But as I watched in my side view mirror, the door of the cruiser opened and I saw two blue stripes. It was a state trooper.

I had been drinking, but I thought I was okay. After the license and registration routine, I walked a straight line. The officer told me I had done real well, and then he asked me to recite the alphabet. That took me by surprise, and, of course, I screwed it up. He took me to the trooper barracks just outside of town, and the breathalyzer showed I was a couple points over the legal limit of .15. I had been driving under the influence.

The young officer asked, "Do you have anyone you could call to drive you home?"

By this time, it was almost three o'clock in the morning. I told him I really wouldn't want to wake anyone up, and he said, "Then you'll spend the night in the county jail."

I said, "Give me a phone. I'll call someone."

The next thing I knew, I was getting into the police car, thinking they were hauling me off to jail. But they were actually driving me home. The next morning I went to my friend's office in town. He was an attorney, and also managed our softball team. I wanted to see if he could do anything to keep me from losing my license. I told him what had happened, and he said there was nothing he could do about it. He suggested I take my medicine like a man. I prepared to walk for ninety days.

Knowing I was going to lose my license, I thought I'd better move to Morris County. Anna hadn't returned from wherever she'd gone, and it had been weeks. I had met a cop, Frank Zuk, from Morris County, who lived a block from the bank. He was going through a divorce and had a bedroom available, so I decided to move in with him.

Frank's apartment was a nice two-bedroom, with a large family room and a kitchen downstairs. It was a duplex, and the owners, who lived on the other side, were nice people. I think they liked having a cop living next door.

The day before I was going to move, we had a big snowstorm. Can you guess who showed up at my apartment during the snowstorm? Anna had come back like nothing was wrong. I told her about my ticket, and that I was moving. Then I said we probably needed some more time apart. We spent that night together, but the next morning I packed. I told her she could have everything in the apartment, and that I'd keep in touch. As usual, I only took my clothes and my fishing equipment.

◆   ◆   ◆

Frank was also into sports, and we played softball on the same team. As an undercover cop, he was working weird hours, and he was hardly ever home. Frank had treated his wife badly. She wasn't a very attractive woman, and he'd told me once told me that he'd been with someone else on his honeymoon. Needless to say, Frank's divorce had gotten messy, and his wife wasn't too pleased that he let me move in. The day I met her, she showed up at the apartment and started banging things around in the kitchen. Then she asked me to please leave for a while, so I went to a nearby tavern for a drink or two.

After his divorce, Frank had his wedding ring made into a pinky ring, so that he would never forget his so-called marriage and would never do it again. He also made a pledge to himself that he would be with as many women as possible, and during the short time I knew him, he was doing pretty well. He seemed to have a thing for dating girls that I had dated. He used to like to waltz them in front of me as he took them to his bedroom. I never knew why.

One day, after I had moved in with Frank, it rained like all get out. I had invited one of the girls from work out to dinner so I wouldn't have to eat alone. Because of the rain, Anna was having trouble with her car, and she called me because she needed my help. She couldn't find me, but after her car was fixed, she began looking for me.

Anna went to the apartment, and Frank's wife was there. After they talked, Anna wrote me a very nasty note. Basically, she said she knew I was with Maureen and had lied to her. Maureen did work at the bank, but I wasn't having dinner with her. The note was filled with a lot of F-words, which was unlike Anna. I am sure Frank's wife fueled Anna's anger. I kept that note for evidence for awhile, but I eventually lost it.

After six months, Frank and I had an opportunity to rent a house on Lake Hopatcong, one of the largest lakes in New Jersey. The house was a two-bedroom ranch, and the garage had been remodeled into a family room with a wood-burning stove. The house was actually across the street from the lake. We joined the association, so we had access to a fishing dock and a boat ramp. I had wanted to live on a lake since I was a kid, so this house was like a dream come true.

Frank and I bought a great boat for fishing and taking the ladies for rides. It was a seventeen-foot fiberglass V hull, with a fifty horsepower outboard engine. White, with a tan interior, it was clean and in good shape. We purchased it from a fellow cop buddy of Frank's. Saturday mornings, I'd wake up, grab my fishing gear, walk to the boat, and go fishing.

I had neither seen nor heard from Anna in a while, and had no clue where she was. Frank and I were hosting a lot of parties at the lake house, and I always invited Bob Gardner. On more than one occasion, when my mother was there at the same time as Bob, she asked him if he knew where Anna was. He always said he had no idea.

When it was time to trade the old VW, I bought a new 1978 Chevrolet Monte Carlo. One day I went for a ride with my date, Valerie, and decided to show Bob my new car. He had bought a small house on a nice little stream out in the country.

As we pulled into Bob's lane, I noticed a large dog that looked familiar, and a brown Chevrolet Nova. The dog was Fa and the car was Anna's. As I stopped the car, Bob came out, looking pretty nervous. I told him Valerie and I had come to show him my new car. He asked if we wanted to come inside. I wasn't so sure about seeing Anna, but Valerie and I went into the house. Anna was sitting on the couch. I asked Bob if he had any liquor, and took a quick shot of whiskey to calm myself down.

Anna and I went outside to talk. I didn't even ask her what she'd been doing. She seemed concerned that I was going to stick her with some bills, but I told her I wouldn't, and we left it at that. It really didn't bother me that she was with Bob, because I knew he would take good care of her.

But remember, I had tried to get them together earlier. It would've saved a lot of pain and heartache if they had just listened to me then. I heard later that they had gotten married. As I mentioned, whenever I am in New Jersey I make a point to see Bob, but Anna has never been with him. Whatever her reasons, that's okay with me.

◆   ◆   ◆

Shortly after high school, Valerie had married a guy named Jack from Bound Brook and had two boys. After her divorce, we'd dated briefly. Then I hadn't seen her for a long time.

Now I was sharing the lake house with Frank and playing softball four nights a week, three in Morris County and one in Somerville. After the last game of the season, the other guys on the team coaxed me into meeting them at The Old York Inn for a drink.

As I was getting out of my car at the tavern, I heard someone call my name. In the dark I couldn't see anyone, but then, out of nowhere, Valerie jumped into my arms. We went in to have a drink, and I only saw the guys from the team in passing. I spent the rest of the evening talking to Valerie and her mother, who happened to be there, too. She told me that she had met a guy at the hospital where she worked as a respiratory therapist. Anyway, she was married to this guy and they had a son, but she was thinking of leaving him. They had only been married about two years, but their sex life had gotten weird and she thought the guy might be gay.

CHAPTER 7
Instant Family Plus One

After that night at The Old York Inn, Valerie and I spoke on the phone quite a bit. Eventually, she and her husband separated, and we started dating. Her boys, John, Steven, and Brad, the baby, seemed to like me. John was a little younger than Kane.

One day I was out in the yard at the lake house, winterizing the boat with Frank, when Valerie pulled up. She said she had just bought a house down the street. Soon I was spending more time at her lake house than my lake house. We decided to try to become a family, and I moved into her house.

I was still working at the bank in Morristown. Valerie wasn't thrilled with some of my coworkers, and I guess I had given her just cause to feel that way. Over the years, I had been quite friendly with some of the girls. Need I say more? I'm not proud of it, but it happened. I started looking for another job.

As I tell you about this time in my life, I'm sure you're thinking, What a dirt bag this guy is. When I originally told my son, Kane, about my plans to write this book, he said, "Tell all." I told him I would be honest and hopefully not upset anyone. But I find I'm upsetting myself.

I landed a job in a small bank in northern New Jersey, but I quickly realized it wasn't where I wanted to be and resigned. At this point, I found out that Valerie wasn't happy living at the lake and wanted to move back to Somerville. I didn't have anything keeping me at the lake, and I wanted to keep the peace, so I agreed she should sell the lake house. We moved to Bradley Gardens, not far from Somerville, where we rented the house next door to Valerie's mother. Our new home was also just down the street from The Old York Inn.

After being out of work for awhile, I got a call from an ex-coworker from the first bank where I'd worked. He was now the president of a small bank in Raritan and offered me a job as manager of a branch in Hillsborough, the closest town south of Somerville.

Valerie and I decided to get married. We went to see my friend, the attorney, who now was also a judge. We were married in his chambers with my mother and Poppa George as our witnesses. Valerie was very pregnant.

When my second son was born, we named him after my best friend, Mark Manara. Things were going pretty well between Valerie and me. One day, an old friend of mine showed up. George had just moved back to town and needed a job. He was married and living with his in-laws. George was a big, muscular guy, with bushy blond hair. He'd played football on a scholarship for the University of Miami, could be mean if he wanted, and wasn't scared of much.

George had married Nancy, a friend of Jill's and mine. I had been best man at their wedding. He and Nancy had had three kids and then gotten divorced, and he'd left town for a few years.

I invited him into our home because he was a friend. I helped him find work with my father-in-law, framing houses. I also helped him with his finances by getting him a loan through the bank.

I knew George didn't pay child support to Nancy for their three kids. She had married an older guy, and he'd adopted the kids. While they were married, George had a vasectomy, but when he married his second wife, she wanted a baby. George had agreed they would use a sperm donor, and his wife had gone through the procedure. But now they were not getting along. He didn't like his new in-laws and was spending all his free time at my house.

One evening, I telephoned a girl at my old bank in Morristown, just to see how things were going. It was nothing more. Valerie came unglued and accused me of being in love with the girl, which certainly was not the case. The girl was just a friend, but Valerie knew how to push my buttons, and she made me furious. After a lot of yelling and screaming, I was at my wit's end.

The next thing I knew, I'd turned the kitchen table over. Well, as far as Valerie was concerned, I had gone too far. She ordered me to leave the house. I said I would, but only if Mark went with me. She said he wasn't going anywhere with me, but that she would leave and take Mark with her. It was below zero outside, and I had no place to go, but I left without Mark. I was basically living out of my car, homeless before being homeless became popular.

I would go to The Old York Inn to eat dinner and meet friends, and to find a place to stay for a night or two. People would always ask me why George's car was at my house. At first I thought he was there comforting Valerie, but it seemed to go on for a long time, and I found out it was much more.

Soon, George's wife started calling me at work, yelling at me because he was with Valerie. She was as whacked as George was, and I told her I really didn't want to talk to her anymore.

I still needed a place to live. Michael, the bartender at The Old York Inn, needed a place, too. So we rented an apartment together, and, with a lot of help from his mother, we moved in. I made it clear that I would go back to Valerie when she was ready. She usually called me at work for money, and she couldn't understand why I had gotten an apartment. I guess she thought I should keep sleeping in my car.

When we'd been separated for several months, I was at The Old York Inn one night with a girl. After the bar closed, we went out to the parking lot, and I kissed her goodnight. George was leaving my house, going to his mother's, and he saw us. Because she knew Valerie, this girl said she wasn't getting in the middle of anything and was going home. I kidded with her, saying that I would just have to follow her home. I certainly didn't mean it. I did follow her out of the parking lot and down the street, but when she turned to go to her house, I went straight and went home. When George told Valerie the story, he made it sound like he'd seen me naked, doing unbelievable things to this girl. Valerie called her, then me, screaming that I was trying to take advantage of a young girl. She basically accused me of stalking.

Two weeks after that messy episode, the bank sent me to a banking course, and I was in New York City for a couple of days. Valerie called, or maybe I called her, and she said she wanted me back. She admitted to being more than close to George. I knew that, but I still got very upset, and was nearly thrown out of the motel for yelling. We got back together, but I think I was just trying to avoid the third strike of another divorce.

I had been a dad to Valerie's boys for quite a while. John and Steven knew their father, but I had been with Brad since he was a little baby. Brad's father paid Valerie a lot of child support, and his paternal grandparents would come to see him, but at one point, Valerie and I went to Brad's father and tried to convince him to let me adopt Brad. After what happened with Kane, I'm ashamed to admit that we tried. It really didn't matter, though, because Brad's father would not agree.

Shortly after we got back together, the lady that owned the house we were renting notified us that she was selling the house. We weren't in a position to buy it, so we were looking for a place. Valerie found a house in Hillsborough that was owned by an architect named Van Cleef. If the name sounds familiar, it is because of Lee Van Cleef. I think he and the architect were cousins or something.

The house in Hillsborough was an old farmhouse on five acres of land, with five upstairs bedrooms. It also had a kitchen, a breakfast nook, a dining room, a TV room, and three other rooms. It was a great place. There was no way we could afford it, but I negotiated with Mr. Van Cleef. I would mow the grass and keep the swimming pool clean, and we agreed on a rent payment that I thought we could handle. There was a tennis court and a basketball hoop in the backyard. The farmhouse was about one hundred years old. The house, being so old, was insulated with straw, which worked pretty well. But when winter came, we could hear mice running up and down inside the walls. So we got a couple of cats.

The farmhouse had fireplaces in most rooms, but they'd all been closed up. The dining room, which I think was originally the kitchen, had a large hearth-type fireplace. I decided to open it and refinish the hearth, the mantle, and the firewall. The fireplace had been painted several times, then closed for quite a while. When I opened it up, there were dead birds, a pile of owl droppings, and a lot of dirt. After the chimney was cleaned, I had it checked out. It was old, but would still work. I considered putting a wood-burning stove in the opening, but was told I would have to install stainless steel pipe, and it would cost a small fortune. That killed that idea. So I removed all the paint from the hearth, the mantle, and the firebox. I closed the chimney back up. The bricks inside the firebox were very old, and the paint remover made them soft. I cemented in fake bricks, and after I was done, it really looked nice.

I mentioned the owl droppings. We had a great barn owl. A barn owl eats a mouse whole and regurgitates the bones and fur. You learn some fascinating things living in an old farmhouse.

The farmhouse itself was a great place for the kids. There was a lot of room to run around, and we had a dog and several cats. The yard was a good place to teach the boys to play basketball, baseball, and football. Of course, Valerie and I were not getting along, which made things difficult at times.

Money wise, things were pretty tight. I was working at the bank, and Valerie was staying home with Mark. She had a job at a doctor's office for one day, but quit that same day. The first summer was okay, and we were able to make the rent payment. But during the winter, with the high heating costs, we couldn't do it. My mother helped us, and we made it through our first, and only, winter at the farmhouse. I spent my vacation time working for my friend, Bob Bocchino. He owned a landscaping company, and he was good enough to put me to work for a week or two at a time.

I tried to teach the boys to fish, but my patience wore thin, and I don't think they really enjoyed it. Steven was the only one who showed much interest. As far as sports, besides playing with the kids, I did nothing. Once, when I asked Valerie if I could play softball, she said she'd rather have me around the house. That was that!

At work, I had been promoted to Director of Marketing and was managing the main branch in the town of Raritan. When I asked the president if the bank would pay for schooling, he said yes. I enrolled in the Graduate School of Retail Bank Management at the University of Virginia in Charlottesville, Virginia. It was a three-year correspondence course, including two weeks a year on campus.

The campus was beautiful, and we stayed in dorms not far from the old football stadium. The original dorms still housed special seniors, who had been selected to reside there. I had the good fortune of seeing the room used by Edgar Allan Poe. Besides attending daily classes, we had time to explore the campus and Charlottesville. We learned about Mr. Jefferson, the school's founder, a man who was well ahead of his time. We even took a Saturday trip to see Monticello.

The bank was going through some changes. My friend, the president, had been replaced, and one stockholder now owned the majority of the bank's stock. He was half African-American, and when he was a young man he had had an idea, but needed some money to get started. He'd come into the bank and asked for a loan. The officer he talked to basically laughed in his face. As he left the bank, he vowed that someday he would own it. As it turns out, his idea was pre-fabrication, and he became very wealthy and bought the bank. He was a very interesting man, and I liked him. His son and I worked together on some design changes for one of the bank's branches, and we got along quite well.

After owning the bank for a short time, he decided to sell, probably for a nice profit. Of course, the new parent bank was much larger, and they had their own marketing person. I still thought I would be kept on as the branch manager, but they fired all senior management. It was the first time in my life that I had been fired or let go from a job, and I was devastated. I was also through with my schooling in Virginia.

Valerie and I had separated just before I lost my job. With the problems at work, and Valerie's constant harping, I'd become so paranoid that I woke up every morning thinking she was mad at me for something. Then I found out that the operations manager at the bank had edged me out for the branch manager's position. I think my multiple sclerosis, or MS, symptoms became worse because of my mental state. In addition to the numbness in my legs, I began having a lot of balance problems.

Valerie moved to an apartment and started babysitting to earn money. I moved into a house with the bartender, Mike, from The Old York Inn. He was living with his girlfriend, who'd been married before and had a beautiful home. It was a split-level on a large lot in Bridgewater. The neighborhood was very upscale, and a couple other guys were renting rooms, too.

The bank had given me a small amount of severance pay. I went on a few interviews, but my only job offers were for work in Newark and New York City. I really didn't want to work either place, so I spent a lot of time at The Old York Inn and saw Kane as often as I could. But my old buddy Michael, the bartender, liked to party, and so did I. And we did party, probably too much.

One day my mother called from Colorado. She had moved there shortly after Poppa George passed away and was willing to send me a ticket to fly to Colorado and find a job. Her offer sounded pretty good, so I took it. I flew to Colorado for a week or two and went to several interviews. My mother said I could live with her and she would help me financially. I had the feeling that she wanted me in Colorado with her and Chip. Once again, the offer sounded really good, so I flew back to New Jersey, planning to pack my belongings in my Chevy Monte Carlo and drive to Colorado.

CHAPTER 8
Head West, Young Man

I said my goodbyes and headed off to Colorado, eager to get started. It was early winter, and I hoped I wouldn't encounter any bad weather. What a trip! Near Omaha, I hit a snowstorm. It was more like a blizzard. The old Monte Carlo didn't have the best traction. The road was slippery, but at least I could see about five car lengths ahead. However, whenever an 18-wheeler passed, the snow would fly, and I couldn't even see the front of my car. I held my breath that the car ahead of me wouldn't stop. Several hours of that got old, and being alone made it worse, especially when the only thing on the radio was country western music.

Exhausted, I rolled in to Lincoln, Nebraska, and spent the night. The next morning was clear and sunny, so I set off again for Colorado. I got to Colorado Springs a day and a half later. Quite the ride!

My mother had a two-bedroom apartment on the north side of Colorado Springs, not far from my brother's home. I went searching for a job but didn't get much response. My brother had lived in the Springs for some time and knew a lot of people. One of his friends offered me a job in his nightclub as a bartender and bouncer. The bartending I knew about, but the bouncing was something new and interesting. Fortunately, I wasn't alone very often. My partner, Doug Yetter, was six feet six inches and 280 pounds. His reputation preceded him.

The nightclub had been a Western bar before Chip's friend bought it. He tried unsuccessfully to turn it into a rock-and-roll sports club. The place was called The Sports Complex. But he soon found out the truth: once a western bar, always a western bar. Finally, he buckled under the pressure and catered to the local cowboys. They were a rough crowd, but Doug knew how to handle them.

I didn't realize how much Colorado was still like the Old West. One night, I was talking to the female bartender, just kidding around. I don't remember what I said, but when I looked up, she was pointing a cute little pearl-handled revolver at me. It really shocked me, but Doug just laughed.

Doug looked like a cowboy, and I started dressing that way, too. I had the hat, shirts, jeans, and boots, but when the fighting started, I would yell for Doug and he would take care of things.

One day I was alone at the club, and a girl and two guys were sitting at a table. All of a sudden the two guys began fighting, and glass started breaking. I rushed over to break it up, grabbed one of guys, and started walking him toward the door. He was a Native American with long black hair, taller than me. Halfway to the door, he swung at me and hit me on the chin. I flinched, but kept walking him out the door. I survived after a stiff drink. He came in later and apologized.

About this time my mother decided she wanted to go to Barbados, and asked me to go with her. I really didn't want to go, but she said she would pay for everything. It was another offer I couldn't refuse.

It was the middle of January, 1982, a good time to get out of cold Colorado and into warm Barbados. Mom and I took a flight from Denver to Miami. We spent the night in Miami before our flight to Barbados. Early the next day, we were on a big silver bird, flying over a lot of ocean. I don't remember how long the flight lasted, but there weren't many of us on the plane. Near the end of the flight, my mother and I decided to have a few cocktails. When we finally landed in Barbados, Mom and I were feeling no pain.

We went through customs and grabbed a taxi to the hotel, a high-class place on the beach called Cobbler's Cove. When we got to the hotel, we checked in and headed for the bar. Some other American guys were there, planning to go for a run in the morning, and I asked them to call me so I could go with them. Fortunately, they recognized the state I was in, and I thanked them later for not waking me.

Naturally, I had my deep-sea rod with me. There was water there, and I was going to fish. I would go to the concrete pier not far from the hotel and throw a lure or two. I only caught a few garbage fish, which I gave to the local kids. I guess they ate them.

The hotel itself was very nice. My mother and Poppa George had stayed there many times before, so Mom knew most of the staff and the manager. My mother and I would have breakfast on our balcony and dinner in the open dining room near the beach, where we could listen to the ocean roll in.

The guests included English folks, Germans, and a few Americans. I met a girl from New York City. Gina was there with her younger sister and their grandparents. She was studying photography in the city. She was twenty-one and I was thirty-two, but we got along just fine. We had a little romance, but nothing too serious.

There were also a couple of sisters from England staying at the hotel. I heard they were quite wealthy. One was tall and good-looking, while the other was a little on the plump side. She was cute and friendly, and I talked to her several times. The tall, good-looking sister was standoffish and wouldn't have much to do the rest of us.

One morning, I was having my coffee on the balcony, and the English girls' apartment was in front of me, off to the right. I looked up from my newspaper and saw the tall sister in a towel, like she just gotten out of the shower. She stood there with her back to me, then dropped the towel. The same thing happened every morning for three days. When I didn't see her one morning, I asked where she was. Her sister told me that she'd left for Australia. Too bad. I really looked forward to our rendezvous every morning.

One night, Gina and I met a couple from England at the neighboring hotel's bar. They were about my age. He was an airline captain, and she was a flight attendant. They said they were married, but I had my doubts. He kept hitting on Gina. His so-called wife was a knockout, and we got along marvelously.

When they said they were leaving, they invited Gina and me to come to their hotel for lunch. I thought it would be a nice gesture to bring a bottle of champagne to the lunch, so I ask the hotel bartender to recommend one.

"Do you want the low price, the medium price, or the high price?" he asked. I told him the medium price would be fine, and to have it chilled so I could pick it up about noon. When I went to get it, I just signed for the champagne without looking at the bill.

Several days later, my mother asked me how the champagne was. I told her it was okay, but nothing special. She informed me that it should have been special, since it cost $175! She was not too happy with me, but she got over it, and it's become a good family story.

I wrote the Brits a few letters after we left Barbados, and she called me several months after I was back home in Colorado. She had a flight to Phoenix, and wanted to know if I would meet her there. Sadly, I was in New Jersey on business, so I missed her call, but my mother took the message.

Our Barbados trip resulted in another family story, too. One night, dinner at our hotel was a buffet, which included some sort of curried meat. As I went through the line I spied some Tater Tots, a familiar food from home, so I grabbed a bunch and sat down to eat. As I bit into one, I discovered it was not a potato, but a fried banana. I was appalled and yelled out to Gina, "Look out for the Tater Tots." Every time I tell that story, I sing the Barbados song, which goes like this: <u>Beautiful, beautiful Barbados, gem of the Caribbean Sea.</u> Now, whenever we have Tater Tots that story has to be told, it is tradition.

With only a week left in beautiful Barbados, my mother and I traveled into the capital city of Bridgetown. We did some shopping and walked down by the mooring docks. As we were walking on the dock, we passed a beautiful two-masted schooner. It was docked pretty close, so I looked in the porthole. And there was a woman with her back to me, naked as a jaybird. I didn't want to look like a pervert or a peeper, so I only looked for a second. Or two.

During the trip, I began to notice I was having trouble walking on the pebbles on the beach when I was bare footed. One day, as I was going into a small town not far from the hotel, I tried to jump over a low stone wall. I made it over the wall, but landed on my butt. I didn't think much of it, just laughed and muttered to myself about being a world-class athlete.

When it was time to say goodbye to Gina and beautiful Barbados, we promised to write. I remember writing to her at least once, but I never heard from her again.

After two weeks in Barbados, I returned to my job at the nightclub. The place was gone, leveled to the ground, and my brother's friend was opening a new nightclub east of town. This guy also managed a softball team, and Chip and I played for one season with him. My brother pitched and I caught, and we won the league that year.

Unfortunately, my MS symptoms were getting worse. Besides the balance problems and the numbness, something new was going on. My legs were not going where I wanted them to, so I was having a hell of a time trying to run. My running didn't hurt me, but it hurt anyone watching. The coach was afraid to let me play. He knew something was wrong, and so did I, but I ignored all my symptoms and went on with my life.

My job search began again. The apartment complex happened to be looking for a manager. I applied and got the job. The position included free rent for Mom. I received minimum wage of about three bucks an hour to collect rents, do simple maintenance and lawn care. The apartment complex was small. It included 4 buildings and a total of 32 apartments. There was a very interesting group of tenants. The complex located in a nice part of the Springs. Most apartments had a great view of Pikes Peak. The rent was not cheap, but they were not the most expensive in the area.

I enjoyed the work specially taking care of the lawn. There happened to be a few single girls renting apartments. I got to know them and dated several.

◆　　　◆　　　◆

Since I'd moved to Colorado, I'd been sending Valerie child support for Mark. I was determined that what had happened with Kane was never going to happen with Mark. Each year, Kane and Mark came to Colorado for visits.

I started hanging out at the new nightclub when it was finished. It was called The Alumni, and pretty much the same people who worked at the old club worked at the new one. The owner's nickname was Jocko, his real name was Bill McMillan. I wasn't asked to work at the new club, I guess Jocko was not impressed by my bartending or bouncing skills. I did go there quite often. It became my place to go.

One night, I was sitting at the corner of the bar, minding my own business and enjoying a nice rum and Coke. Two girls walked by, but I really didn't pay much attention to them. When they sat down, the girl nearest to me kicked my leg. She quickly apologized, and we started to talk. She was a petite little thing, and cute, with short blond hair. It never fails that when you're not looking for anyone, you find her. Donna managed a large apartment complex. So we had something in common.

Donna and I started to date. We had some fun, if you know what I mean. Donna taught me a lot about women and their sexual needs and wants. She certainly wasn't shy, and she spoke her mind. I only wished someone had told me years earlier what I learned from her.

My mother was not happy because I was spending too much time at Donna's place. My mother was receiving all the complaint calls from the complex's tenants. Do you believe that she wanted me home to answer complaints rather than me being at Donna's having fun? Like, what was she thinking? I'm only kidding. I did go home and took care of the complaining tenants.

Chip had been financing automobiles for a Chevrolet dealership for some time. He knew a lot of people in the business, and when he found out that the Pontiac dealership was looking for a finance man, he suggested I apply. We thought that me being in the banking business I should be qualified. I knew all about auto loans and credit insurance. I went in, interviewed, and got the job and resigned from the apartment complex. The pay at the dealership was pretty good, much more than minimum wage.

It was a two-man operation, and my boss seemed to be sick a lot. I ended up doing most new work myself, without much training. I was easily working ten to twelve hours a day, and sometimes more. The long hours and stress were not good and were taking their toll on me. I started to sweat profusely. It became so bad that I would stuff folded paper towels in the arm pit of my under shirt. I also became short tempered. I know now, that MS was the cause of these strange happenings.

They gave me a new Pontiac Grand Prix to drive. It was fully equipped and all leather. Donna really like it. Then one day, during a big meeting, the owner told all the salespeople they weren't getting paid because of the finance department. As usual, my boss was out sick that day. After the meeting, I lost my temper and said a few things I probably shouldn't have. The next day I was called to the manager's office and fired. They had the gall to drive me home in my demo. All the sweating and tamper stuff were gone once I was home. Once again, I was unemployed.

A day after losing my job, I was looking out the window of Donna's apartment, and I knew something just wasn't right. After several minutes, I realized I was having double vision. I drove home with one eye shut and decided I'd better go see an eye doctor. After a thorough examination, the eye doctor, Dr. Tom Wilson, told me that there was nothing wrong with my eyes and I should see a neurologist.

I picked a neurologist, Dr. Olivera, from the phone book, and made an appointment. My mother went with me and waited outside while I saw the doctor. By this time, the double vision was gone, but when I told Dr. Olivera all my symptoms, he did a short examination and told me I had multiple sclerosis. I didn't know what that was, and the first thing I asked was whether it would affect my sons in any way. The doctor said there was no evidence of it being hereditary.

He gave me a couple of brochures about multiple sclerosis, said that I was still pretty strong, and told me that unless I had pain, there was no need to see him again. As we left, my mother asked what was wrong with me.

"I have MS," I said.

She said, "I know you're a mess, but what's really wrong?" We laughed and I handed her a brochure. My mother was a great lady.

I suppose it was a relief after so many years, to finally know what was really wrong with me. Dr. Olivera had told me not to tell my employers about my diagnosis. He said people just didn't understand the disease. I had never heard of multiple sclerosis, but the brochures he gave me explained a lot.

This disease affects the nervous system. The central nervous system [CNS] is made up of two main parts, the spinal cord and the brain. The CNS receives nerve impulses from all parts of the body, and then sends out appropriate responses to the body's muscles and organs.

Nerve fibers in the brain, spinal cord and optic nerves are surrounded by a myelin sheath. This insulating layer of myelin helps nerve impulses travel more quickly (similar to the way in which plastic insulates electrical wiring to make electrical conduction faster).

MS affects the CNS by damaging the myelin sheath. Myelin is lost in multiple areas, leaving plaques or scars called sclerosis. This damage or loss of myelin can prevent nerve signals from being conducted, or can cause those signals to be conducted too slowly.

Multiple sclerosis is an unpredictable disease that can follow several different courses. Throughout the course of MS, symptoms can occur in relapses. A relapse (also known as a flare-up, attack or exacerbation) is a recurrence of a neurological symptom or symptoms that typically lasts for several days to several weeks. Relapses occur from time to time throughout the course of multiple sclerosis. Although the course of MS varies, the disease tends to take one of the following forms:

1. RELAPSING-REMITTING. People with relapsing-remitting MS experience attacks that can last days or weeks. Following these attacks, symptoms may lessen dramatically or disappear completely before returning.

2. PRIMARY-PROGRESSIVE. This form of MS is characterized by symptoms that progressively worsen over time. There are generally no remissions, though symptoms might temporarily improve.

3. SECONDARY-PROGRESSIVE. For some patients, MS initially follows a relapsing-remitting course that later changes to a secondary-progressive course.

4. PROGRESSIVE-RELAPSING. Less than 5% of the MS population experience progressively worsening symptoms accompanied by acute attacks.

5. BENIGN. People with this form of MS tend to experience numbness and blurred vision during attacks. Symptoms generally do not worsen. The disease follows this course in approximately 20% of people diagnosed with MS.

I told Donna about my diagnosis. At first she was very supportive and we continued to date for a short time. I didn't have a job and money was tight. One day Donna came to see me and told me not to call her until I found another job. I thought, Boy, that was cold.

As far as the disease was concerned, I read everything I could find. I knew it could get better, stay the same, or get worse. I refused to consider the third possibility. I'd been assured that I wasn't going to die soon, and I didn't expect to suffer. I always felt fortunate that it wasn't cancer. Things could have been worse, right? I was in denial, again.

One day, the girls at The Alumni said they'd heard of a talent agency who was looking for a cowboy for an advertising campaign, and they suggested that I go and interview. It was for a cigarette company ad. You know the one, with the cowboy smoking? The girls thought I was a shoe-in to get the job. The hundred-thousand-dollar-a-year salary sounded pretty good, too. I put on my best Cowboy garb, hat and all, and went to the interview. I had never seen so many cowboys and cowgirls in one place. I finally got to the interview and the interviewer asked me to show him my hands, he said, "You have banker hands," and I laughed. They were looking for the rugged type, like a real cowboy not a drugstore cowboy. It was the old story, don't call us we will call you.

Jock's wife, Lynne, had also interviewed, but for the cowgirl job. Since Jocko was always at the bar so was Lynne. I talked to her a lot. She was absolutely stunning, with long dark hair, a beautiful face and a perfect shape. She was picked to go to the second interview in Dallas. Jocko being a very jealous person, told her that she could not go. It would have been neat to see her in commercials. Not long after this, Jocko and Lynne got divorced. I think Jocko had been married six or seven times.

On the way home from the talent agency, I stopped at the dealership to see Chip. I hung around, talked for a couple of hours, and met the owners. The next day my brother called and said Mr. Williams, one of the owners, wanted to see me. He offered me a job in the finance department on a trial basis. I took him up on his offer, and Chip, Paul Dally, and I became the finance department.

The dealership was family-owned and operated. In addition to Mr. Williams, there was his sister, Charlotte, her husband, Paul McDonnell, and their son, Michael, who was the corporate attorney. It was a great place to work.

After a short trial period, Mr. Williams hired me and sent me to insurance school in Dallas. Credit life and disability insurance was not new to me, because I had sold insurance at the bank.

One day, at the dealership I was having a heck of a time coming down the stairs from a meeting. Mrs. McDonnell asked me what was wrong. I had to be honest and told her about my diagnosis. Later, she came to me and said, "No matter what happens, as long as you can get to work and do, you have a job. You need not worry about working for Williams Chevrolet. That was really nice to know, because not long after that I started using a wheelchair to get around.

Paul Dally, our boss, was a kick. He entertained the customers, making them laugh while he sold them insurance and financed their car. We had loads of fun and made a whole lot of money.

I had been working at Williams Chevrolet for a couple of months when I received a phone call from Donna. She had heard that I was back at work and she wanted to meet me at The Alumni. The way she dumped me, I wanted to talk to her. I met her that night at The Alumni. She started talking to me like we had never broken up. I listened and then with one single hand motion with one finger, she knew how I felt. She got up off her stool and ran out of the building.

I started to feel real bad for what I did. When I got home I called her and apologized, but we never went out together again. On several occasions I would see her in different places. She was cordial and we would say hello.

I had been talking with Valerie, at night from the club, about her and the boys moving out to Colorado. I was making enough to support them, so she decided to come, and I rented a house not far from the dealership. She drove a loaded U-Haul to Colorado, a pretty gutsy trip with three kids. John, her oldest son, stayed with his father in New Jersey and flew out later. So, we all moved into the rented house, and we put the boys in school. I thought things were going pretty well. We had a few money problems, but nothing serious.

Only about a month later, I came home from work to find a loaded U-Haul in the driveway, and Valerie announced she was going back to New Jersey. Then she told me she had talked to my mother, and it would be okay if I moved back to Mom's apartment. Valerie and the boys left, but around 11:00 p.m., I got a phone call. She had made a wrong turn in Wyoming and asked if I wanted her to come back. I said no, and I was on my own again. I moved back to my mother's and started hanging out at The Alumni.

One day, I got a call from Valerie and she said she had just seen a show on TV about a new trial for multiple sclerosis that was being conducted in New York. She gave me all the information, and I sent for an application. After some time, I got a long, involved application to fill out and return. Several months had passed when I received a letter saying that I was a candidate for the trial and had an appointment at the hospital in New York. I called my uncle Phil and asked if he would let me stay at his house and drive me to the hospital. Of course, he said yes.

I was still working for Williams Chevrolet, and when Mr. Williams and the salesmen found out I needed to go to New York, they generously got together and bought me a plane ticket. Several months later, I flew to New Jersey. One of the stipulations of the trial was that you still had to be walking. I was, but I needed a cane because my condition had gotten worse.

It was January 1984 when my uncle drove me to Albert Einstein Hospital in the Bronx for the interview. I walked into the interview room, but it was quite a distance, and I was exhausted. I met with a young neurologist, who asked a lot of questions before he examined me. After the examination, he told me I wasn't qualified to be included in the trial. When he asked what my neurologist was doing for me, I told him that my neurologist said I didn't need to see him unless I had pain. That young doctor sat me down, told me to find a new neurologist, and sent me home.

When I deplaned in Colorado Springs, I needed a wheelchair. I made an appointment with a different neurologist, Dr. Richard Bell, who told me there were several things we could do to try to help me. The first thing he wanted to do was put me in the hospital.

CHAPTER 9
A New Beginning:
Life Can Be Good

The day I had to report to the hospital, my mother and Uncle Bill were going to drive me to Penrose Hospital. I remember having one hell of a time getting down the stairs of the apartment. I went down the steps on my butt. My legs just would not work. Fortunately, we had the wheelchair.

When we got to the hospital, they were doing construction on the rehab floor, so they put me in a room on the tenth floor. I didn't have to use the wheelchair much, but needed my cane to get to the bathroom. The bathroom was not wheelchair accessible. In a hospital?

Now here's the part of my story that I consider the greatest love story ever told, at least for me. But first of all, let me assure you that I had no desire to meet anyone. I was in that hospital to get better.

As I sat in my wheelchair at the nurses' station, someone came from behind me, saying my name. She pronounced it wrong, and I corrected her. I looked at her nametag, which said Kathleen M. Groeger. I pronounced it as it was spelled, Groeger, and she told me it was pronounced Gregger.

She was my physical therapist. She was a cute young lady, short blondish hair, an athletic shape. You could just tell she was a strong lady. I've always said that I had a thing for her that very second. I had physical therapy Monday through Friday and was getting my ACTH treatments, too. I was still walking with my cane. Dr. Bell assured me that these treatments were going to do some good. He and I got along great, because he was also a fisherman.

Then Saturday came, and there was no Kathleen. She had gone to a class in Denver for the weekend, and I had another therapist. I felt abandoned. Dr. Bell had said he would discharge me on Monday, but I asked him if I could stay a couple extra days. I did tell him I wanted to see Kathleen again. Dr. Bell granted my request, so I got to see her a couple more times.

On the last day, she came in to see me, but I was asleep. She left a note with some exercises on it and her home phone number, saying that if I needed anything, to give her a call.

I was discharged from the hospital feeling pretty strong. I had to stay at Chip's house, because my mother's apartment had too many stairs. My brother had some friends from New Jersey, Mel and Kathy, staying with him. I really wanted to call Kathleen, but I was a little hesitant. I was 10 years older than her and she was in a whole different place than me. The story is will I drag her to me or will she lift me to her? I talked to Kathy for some time about the situation. She told me I didn't have anything to lose, and that I should call. We all had plans to go out to dinner, so I thought it would be a great time to invite Kathleen, too.

When I called and invited her to dinner, Kathleen said she couldn't date a patient. I told her I wouldn't be her patient anymore, and she agreed to go to dinner with us. It wasn't like we were going to be alone. We went to a great restaurant called Zeb's, named for Zebulon Pike, as in Pike's Peak. We all had a good time.

I invited Kathleen to The Alumni for drinks after dinner, and she accepted. She said she was not a bar person. I assured her that it was a very nice place. When we entered The Alumni, she was walking and I was riding. Despite the hospitalization and the treatments, I was getting worse. I asked Kathleen to stop before we went into The Alumni, and said, "Let's get this over with now, so that we don't have to worry about it the rest of the night." I kissed her right on the lips. I had never tried that approach before, honest! But it worked.

That night at my brother's, we talked, and we talked, and we talked. I found out that Kathleen was one of fourteen children and that her father was a doctor. Kathleen was the twelfth child and, of course, was a physical therapist.

All the Groeger kids are all successful in their own right. Mom and dad raised eight girls and six boys. There is not a slacker in the whole group. The oldest boy is a vascular surgeon in California. Lynne, the oldest girl in the Groeger family, was three months and eleven days older then me. She is good-looking, but so are all the Groeger girls. When she was five years old, she had gotten polio. She wears a brace, walks with a limp, and uses wooden crutches occasionally. The polio never stopped her from doing anything. I think Kathleen became a physical therapist because of Lynne, who's an unbelievable lady. She is a physician's assistant, and I was told that when she took the test, she earned the highest score in the nation. She started, and runs, a clinic up in the mountains where she lives.

There is also another doctor, a family practice physician in South Dakota, a medical transcriptionist in the Springs, a successful jeweler in Texas, a manager of a molybdenum mine in the Colorado Mountains, a retired county worker who knows and can do everything, an artist and heart therapist in town, an elementary school teacher in California, a supervisor for a large paving company in Florida, a manager of a prosthesis and brace company in the Springs, a chemical engineer and wife and mother with three successful local businesses with her husband, an electrical engineer and wife and mother living up Ute Pass. There's not a drug addict or an alcoholic in the bunch.

They are all wonderful, talented people, but I do have to make special mention of two brother-in-law's: the retired county worker. Dennis is two years older than I am. As I said, he knows everything and can do everything. Several years back he was diagnosed with MS. He has been taking Avonex and is doing well, but tires easily and has a problem with his short-term memory. As a county worker, he ran heavy equipment and was forced to retire because of MS. Everyone loves Uncle Dennis. Uncle Bob my hero. Bob was married early in life and had three beautiful children. The kids were young when their mother took them and left Bob. Their mother wanted a different kind of life. Within a short period of time, Bob had custody of all three kids. Bob's main purpose in life was the three kids. Jessica, Nick and Jackie grew up to be great people. All three graduated from college. Bob without a concern for his needs or wants the kids came first. Not like me, who always thought of himself first, Bob took the high road. With eight sisters he had some help. Aunt Lynne was always available for Bob and the kids. The kids are all grown with lives of their own. I recently told Bob that it is Bob's time. So, any lady looking for a GREAT guy, he is available.

Kathleen's brothers and sisters are spread out over the West and we really don't see all of them often. On special occasions, like mom's eightieth birthday all the siblings were together.

The night we met, Kathleen and I found out that we generally had the same ideals and thoughts about life. She had recently graduated from physical therapy school and had her undergraduate degree in psychology. She played soccer and softball, and in high school held the school record for the shot-put.

Well educated, pretty, and athletic, too. What more could I ask for? When Kathleen invited me home to Woodland Park, I met her parents and one of her seven sisters. She told me later that her sister said anyone like me was either married or had been married. How right she was. I knew that I would have to be up front with Kathleen and tell her my whole story.

Kathleen had invited me to watch her play soccer. On our way to the game we stopped by Prospect Lake, and I told her I had something to tell her. I thought if I told her something horrible first, the truth wouldn't seem so bad. So I told her I was gay and had herpes.

That shocked her, and I decided I'd better tell her the truth before she started to believe the lies. So I told her I had been married three times, had two children, and wasn't actually divorced yet. She said that the divorce would have to be finalized for her to see me. She also said that she would not have sex until she was married, and she wouldn't marry anyone she hadn't known for at least a year. Believe it or not, I told her that wasn't a problem.

Kathleen said she would not marry a smoker, and I was smoking at that time. I promised her that I'd quit and that I would finalize the divorce from Valerie as soon as possible, which I did.

We started dating and saw each other every night after work. We went to dinner at Red Lobster, or some other nice restaurant in town, at least four times a week. We were really getting along and enjoyed each other's company. We'd gone fishing a few times in the mountains, and Kathleen was a great sport.

I decided to buy a fifteen-foot Crestliner with an open bow and a fifty-horsepower outboard motor. The boat also had a trolling motor and plate. She was orange and white, with a canopy and covers for the front and back, plus the full mooring cover. Kathleen and I would pack up Friday night and go fishing until Saturday afternoon. We did this twice a month or more during the summer. I named the boat My Kat'leen, and had it spelled out on both sides of the boat. Kathleen got a big kick out of that.

The first time we went fishing with the boat, we went to a local reservoir, Antero Reservoir. I had bought Kathleen a new fishing rod and reel, a very nice spinning outfit. We were drifting along, casting from the boat, and Kathleen was in the front. When I noticed she was sitting down, crying, I asked her what was wrong. She said she had forgotten to hold on to the rod and had cast it into the lake. I told her it wasn't a problem, because I had plenty of rods she could use, and we could replace her outfit. We still laugh about it to this day.

I was pretty much wheelchair-bound by this time. At one point, the doctor put me on Prednisone. I thought he'd cured me. With my Loft-strand crutches, which are also called Canadian crutches, I walked nearly the length of a football field. But the results only lasted a couple days.

I had also bought a full-size, short bed Chevrolet van, with a chair lift and hand controls. The van made things a lot easier, and I could still stand with help and walk for short distances with crutches.

I had met Kathleen in May. It was now November 1984, and we were still getting along very well. I decided to ask her to marry me. I know what you're thinking: <u>Is this idiot going to do it again?</u> I truly thought long and hard about what I was planning. Was I setting myself up for failure for the fourth time? Everything that you're thinking went through my mind, too. But things were different this time. I had never felt this way about anyone before.

I went out and bought a beautiful diamond ring. On Thanksgiving Day, at my mother's apartment, I asked Kathleen to marry me. My mother had the champagne chilled. Kathleen said yes, I gave her the ring, and we drank champagne. Kathleen had said she wouldn't marry anyone unless she'd known him for a year, so when she went home that night, she didn't tell her family about the ring.

The next day she talked to her brother, Bob, who told her to give the ring back. He said if I loved her, I would wait. And the next day she gave the ring back to me, explaining that with my mother there, and the camera and champagne, she hadn't been able to say no. When I told Chip, he said I'd better get rid of the diamond, or it would be bad luck. So I did!

Kathleen and I continued dating. I was still working at Williams Chevrolet. One of the fellows at the dealership dabbled in diamonds, and I bought one, just a diamond with no ring. I gave it to Kathleen for Christmas and told her whenever she was ready, we would build a ring for it. We left it at that.

Sometime in the fall of 1984, I got a call from Paul Franklin, a sportswriter for my hometown daily newspaper. He told me someone wanted to dedicate a football game in my honor. The only two people who knew my diagnosis were Kane and Mark. Of course their mothers also knew. He asked me a lot of questions about how I was doing. I was in shock, but I thought it was a great thing. I found out later that someone was Jill. She told me she had actually done it because I had done a lot for sports in Somerville and also Kane was having an identity problem. She assured me Kane and Mark would both be there.

I asked Kathleen to go with me, and she agreed. So Kathleen, my mother, and I flew to New Jersey for the Friday night game. Somerville was playing Piscataway. I got to sit on the sidelines with my ex-coach, Al "Boomie" Malekoff, my best friend Mark Manara, my Kathleen, Mom, and my two sons. There were a whole bunch of my friends in the stands. I spent the entire game going from the sidelines to the fence, seeing people I hadn't seen in a long time. It sure was a great night, and I'll never forget it.

Saturday morning we went to watch Kane play football for Bernardsville High. Two of my good friends went with us. Mike Trippanera, the bartender at the Old York Inn and Carl Hammerdorfer, the hammer, were two close friends during my turbulent time before I left New Jersey. It was neat to see my boy play. And he was wearing number 86, which had been my number when I played. His team lost, but I won the raffle. We left Sunday because Kathleen and I had to be back at work Monday morning.

Kathleen and I continued to date. She talked quite a bit with her mom and dad. They were both very concerned about my multiple sclerosis. Her dad, being a doctor, knew how the disease could progress. He didn't feel she should work all day with sick people, and then come home and continue working at night. I was appalled by his comments. First, I was still in denial, and second, I had no plans to get worse.

When Kathleen got tired of going up and down the mountain pass, she rented an apartment in Colorado Springs, closer to where I lived. We continued to see each other every day. Then one evening I went to her apartment, and she was cold and aloof. Her father was putting pressure on her to break up with me, so she told me we should stop seeing each other.

I went bonkers and told her to go out and get herself some young buck. She said didn't want a young buck. After a long conversation, she finally told me that I was the one she wanted. The young buck thing still gets a smile from both of us whenever it's mentioned.

I was still doing everything for myself, like getting dressed, taking a shower, shaving, brushing my teeth, and combing my hair. I was only having trouble walking. I could still drive my van and work. I would tell Kathleen, "What do I need to do, just die and blow away? What am I, a piece of wood? I don't matter? I'm a person, too, with feelings." I guess I just loved her so much, I didn't see the whole picture.

One day when I was at physical therapy, a guy from a wheelchair company came in with an ultra-light sports chair called a Quickie. It was dreamed up and designed by a paraplegic. I thought, <u>Who better to design a wheelchair than someone in a wheelchair?</u> I tried it out and thought it was great. I bought it without ever having the chair fitted to me, which I later found out was a big mistake. I could not understand why I felt tired all the time or why my bottom hurt.

Kathleen and I learned a great deal together about wheelchairs, multiple sclerosis, and life in general. Once we found out that the chair was causing my problems, we ordered one the right way. We found an occupational therapist who specialized in fitting people to wheelchairs, and let him do the job. We went through the whole measuring process, and we ordered another Quickie that fit my needs. It took a month for it to come in, but once it did, I really noticed the difference. The new chair wasn't quite as sporty as the first, but it sure was functional and a pleasure to be in.

I also found out that there is nothing worse than the wrong seat cushion. Your butt hurts all day if your cushion isn't doing its job. Considering the length of time you are sitting, you need to make sure it's right.

In late summer of 1986, Kathleen and I were still going strong. I decided to look into building a home. I found a realtor and his wife, who had MS, and they specialized in handicapped-accessible homes. They knew a lot about building a wheelchair-accessible house, and yet, their own home was not.

They took us to a new development in town on the northeastern edge of the Springs. I told Kathleen if we didn't get married, my mother and I would move into the new home, but I needed her help in securing the mortgage. I told her I would put up all the money for the house if she would sign for the mortgage with me. It wasn't a bad deal for her, because she would own half the home without making any financial investment.

The builder, David Keller, was very helpful. His father had been in a wheelchair, so he was very aware of what my needs were. We made a deal to have a ranch model built, and financed the mortgage through the builder's source. Kathleen was very nervous about the whole thing. We would travel to the construction site every Sunday and take pictures of the house. We have quite an album of pictures documenting the process from empty lot to completed home. The house was due to be finished in December 1986.

A month before the completion date, Kathleen came to me and said she had found the perfect setting for our diamond. It was time to go talk to Dr. and Mrs. Groeger.

We had a very good conversation. I think they realized we were very much in love, but, of course, they were trying to protect their child. Being a strong Catholic family, they had a lot of reservations about me. And honestly, with my past, they should have been concerned. But I knew that this relationship was very different from anything I had experienced before. The multiple sclerosis was a big issue with the doctor, which I couldn't understand. I can understand now, but back then, I really couldn't, because the old denial thing was upon me.

Dr. and Mrs. Groeger hesitantly gave us their blessing, but asked me to go through the Catholic Church for an annulment. They didn't realize that there was more than one divorce. I got all the necessary paperwork to apply for the annulments, but filling it out was very difficult for me, and the stress affected me physically. It was very much like the early stages of writing this book.

Kathleen and I explained to her folks about my past and told them we would get married in a Methodist church, with a Catholic priest in attendance. Things were looking pretty good. Kathleen started all the planning for the wedding. Whenever anyone asked how long we'd been dating, I'd say I had chased her for three years, until she finally caught me.

◆　　　◆　　　◆

Right in the middle of our wedding planning, Mr. Williams sold the dealership and retired. Chip left immediately and went to work for the Porsche/Audi dealership in town. Paul and I thought we could handle the department by ourselves. The new owner, a guy from Detroit, owned twelve other dealerships. He sent one of his top men from Detroit to take over this location, and the guy came in and really cleaned house. He didn't like Paul's way of selling, so Paul moved to another Chevrolet dealer in town. If I'd been Paul, I would have left, too.

Several guys were hired to work in the finance department, but the new manager didn't like any of them. One by one, everyone left, until I was the only one there.

I could see the writing on the wall. Just working ten to twelve hours a day wasn't going to get the job done, and although the new owner assured me that he would get more help, he never said who or when. My MS was getting worse again, and under those working conditions, it would be unbearable pretty quickly. I resigned a week before Christmas. Fortunately, I still qualified to receive unemployment. We didn't tell Dr. and Mrs. Groeger, and the wedding plans went ahead.

Kathleen and I signed the mortgage papers on schedule. She would move in right away, we would get married on January 17th, and then I would move in, too. Everything was going along just fine, except that I was unemployed again.

Chip would be my best man. Kathleen's sister Lorie would be her maid of honor. All the invitations were mailed, and reception plans were made. I was in charge of the honeymoon plans, so I made reservations for our wedding night at a classy hotel in town.

On Saturday morning, January 17, 1987, we assembled at the Methodist church for our nuptials. Before Kathleen walked down the aisle, her mother asked if she was really going through with it. Kathleen said yes, and she did.

We had planned that at the end of the ceremony, I would stand and kiss Kathleen. But whenever I stood up, I would have a little gas, so I asked Chip to cough when I was about to stand and kiss Kathleen. He did, and everything went off without a hitch.

We had invited Dr. Bell to come to the wedding, because if it hadn't been for him, we wouldn't have met. He actually showed up, which pleased us both. The reception was held at The Palmer House. We had a buffet dinner with champagne. Kathleen's aunt made us a beautiful cake.

As I was mingling, I heard Paul talking to Dr. Groeger about work, and cringed. Paul was telling the doctor how sorry he was that he couldn't get me a job with his new employer. I breathed a sigh of relief. That wasn't so bad. Unfortunately, we hadn't told Paul that Dr. Groeger didn't know I had quit the dealership. But then I heard him assure my new father-in-law that I shouldn't have any problem finding a job. The situation became a bit tense when the Groegers realized their daughter had just married an unemployed cripple. Fortunately, when Kathleen explained the situation, her parents were somewhat satisfied, and the reception continued smoothly.

After the reception, when everybody was getting into cars to leave, I rolled myself over to the doctor's car. I promised Dr. Groeger I would take care of his daughter. He smiled and nodded, as though he knew I would take care of Kathleen.

Off to the hotel we went. After three years of dating and not having sex, our expectations were pretty high. We won't get into all the details, but we had a great night.

Sunday morning, we couldn't wait to go to our new home, open our wedding gifts, and start our life together. Kathleen had to work Monday morning, so we postponed our honeymoon

go to see a neurologist. Here we go again! I made
an appointment with a doctor -- neurologist -- my
mother and I went to the appointment. After a very
short examination he said I had multiple sclerosis.
The first thing I asked was were my kids in any risk.
He said not that they know of. He also said that I did
not have to come back to him unless I had pain. He
never said change your lifestyle and all the other
things that goes with multiple sclerosis. He gave the
a flyer about multiple stores is. It was kind of a relief
to finely now what all the symptoms were about. On
the layout my mother asked what did the doctor said.
I told her high half drama pass. She said to me that
she knew I was a mass. Hot, hot hot. Ha Ha Ha

It was time to read up on this disease. Which I did
with every book I could find. I thought to myself not
to bad. I still felt pretty good and my eyes side returned.
So, no problem. I felt and was assured that I wasn't
going to die soon and that it wasn't cancer. I thought
I would remain about the same physically and
mentally.
my brother had been working at a Chevrolet
dealership financing automobiles in new a lot of
people in the business. The fact that I had been in
banking in new finance, we set out to get a new job
that would pay. after a few interviews I landed a job
at a Pontiac dealership in the finance department. I

As I've mentioned, this is one of the first pages written that shows
the voice-activated system and how It compares to the final
manuscript. Compare this page with page number 87 of the final
document.

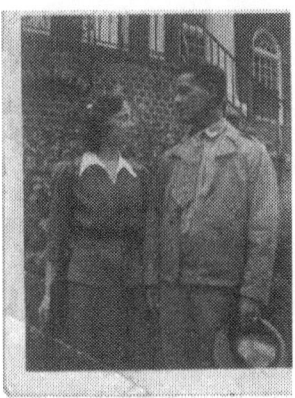

Early picture of the folks

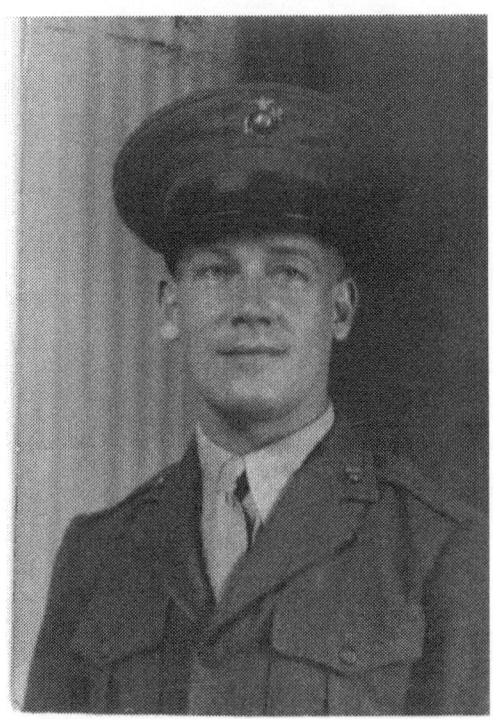

My uncle Bill told me that my father was older than the rest of the recruits. He thought my father wouldn't make the cut at Paris Island. I guess the old man was tougher than he thought.

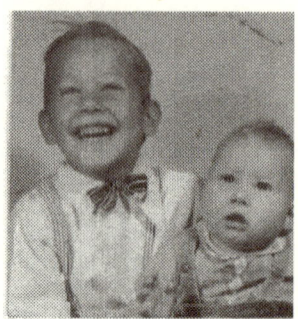

The earliest picture I could find of my brother and me. I am just a baby and I look very confused

Somerville to honor former gridder suffering from multiple sclerosis

By PAUL FRANKLIN
Courier-News Sports Writer

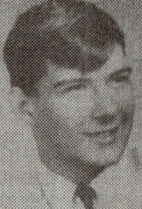

VAN GRAEF
...1967 graduation photo

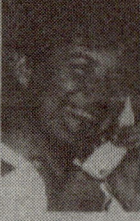

VAN GRAEF
...in Colorado home this year

Continued on Page D-3

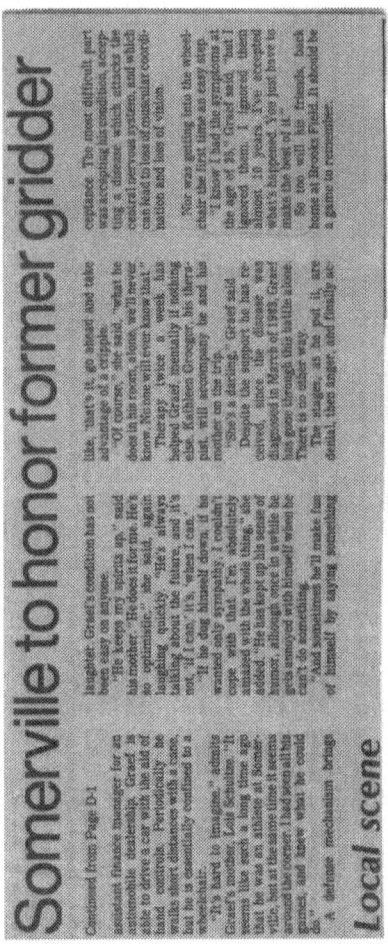

Somerville to honor former gridder

Continued from Page D-1

Local scene

1984 my friends in Jersey found out that I had MS.
The high school decided to have the Piscataway game in my
benefit. A lot of people were there. I did not get a chance to speak
to everyone. I saw people I had seen in years. It was great. This
article mentions how my friends ragged about not playing defense
or being tough. During this exact game in 1966, I did play defense
and I intercepted a pass. But they forget. I may not have been tough
but I could catch the ball. The person who started the whole thing
was Kane's mother, Jill.

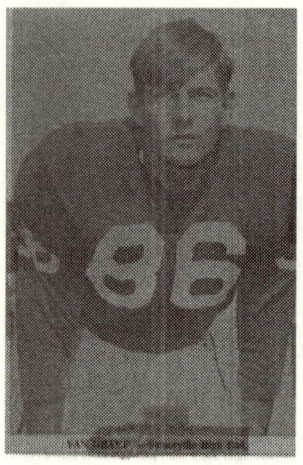

This picture was taking for the booster club and it was also used as my picture for the All County team

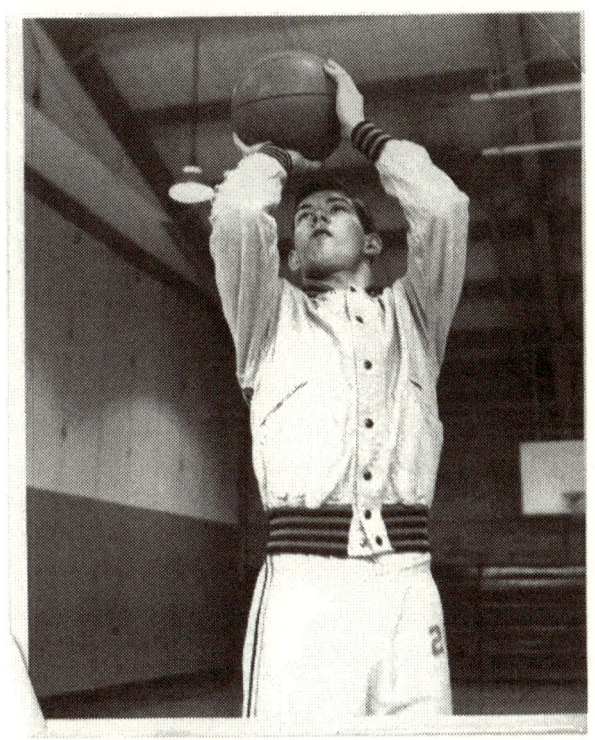

This picture was taken for the all County team

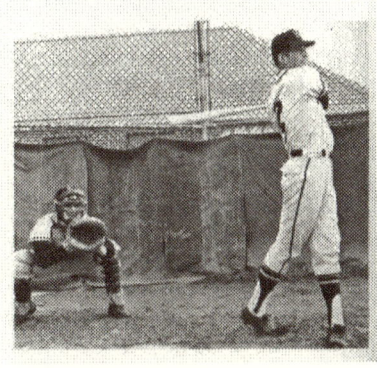

This is the only picture of high school baseball I could find
I hated the picture they took for the all County team

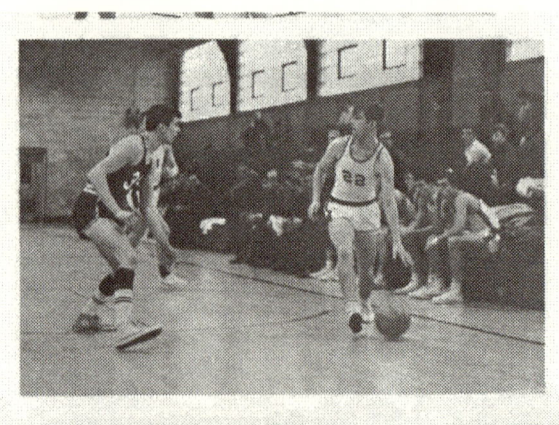

I really like this picture. I believe we were playing Princeton high
school. We did win that game.

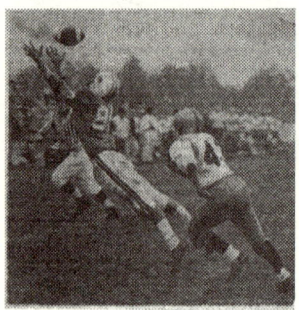

My favorite picture. Mark Manara said I always knew where the
camera was. The real deal is that I was the only one making plays
down field.

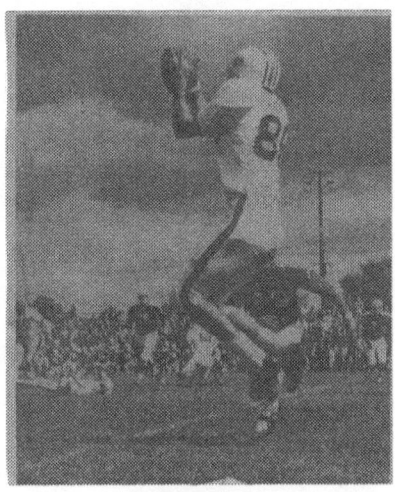

Another catch, I guess Manara was right. I found another camera!

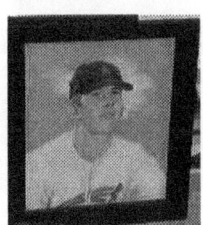

My brother had this painting done when he was with the Houston
Astros
Baseball Club.

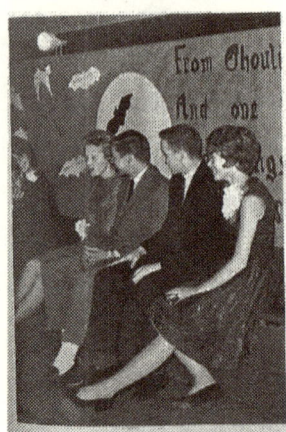

This is interesting! My first date with Jill Neumann, the night I met Penny Nuss. That's Jill on the far left and then me and then Winks and Beverly Overk. Beverly was actually the first girl I ever kissed.

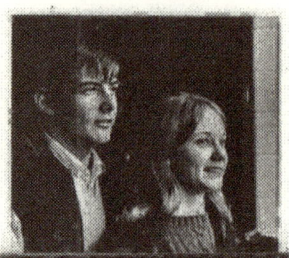

Our senior year, we started dating December third 1966. It was a long way from that freshmen dance.

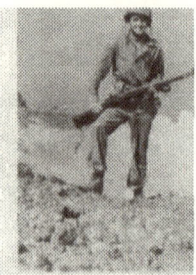

This picture was taken in Iwo Jimo, Mount Surabachi He said that he was cowboying. This was the setting for the raising of the flag.

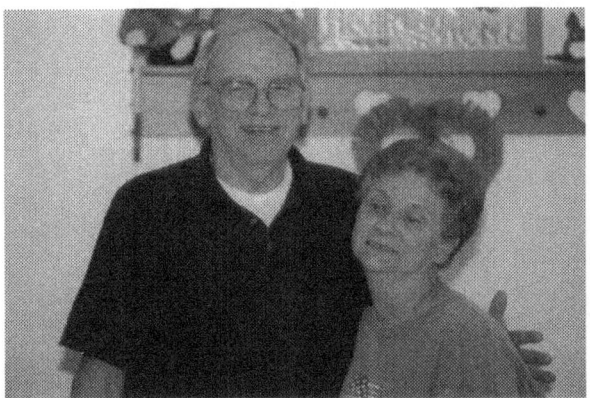

Everyone's favorite aunt and uncle. Specially my kids, Kathleen and I
. I always say that I am their favorite nephew. They will always a big
part of my life.

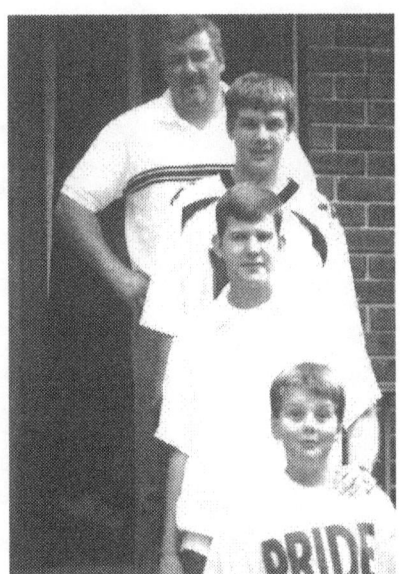

Kane, Ty, Mark, and Tucker I believe this was only the third time all
the boys were together.

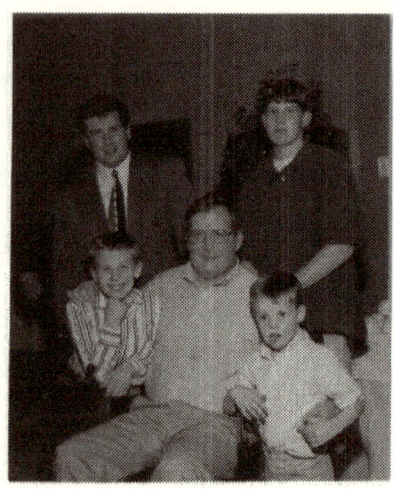

I believe that this is the second time the boys were all together.

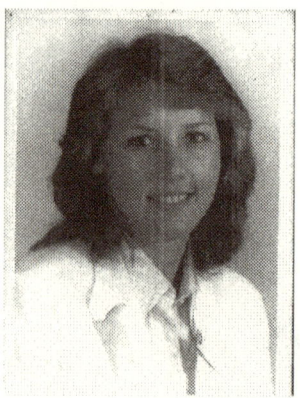

This picture was taken in 1984 shortly after I met Kathleen. She only
has grown more beautiful each day since.

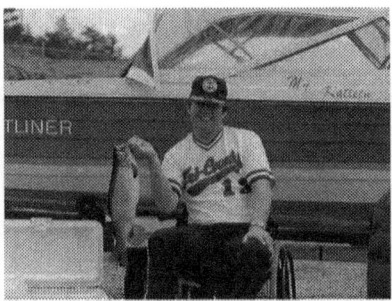

Kathleen and I fishing Spinney Mountain Reservoir. My boat and the beautiful cutthroat trout that now hangs on our living room wall.

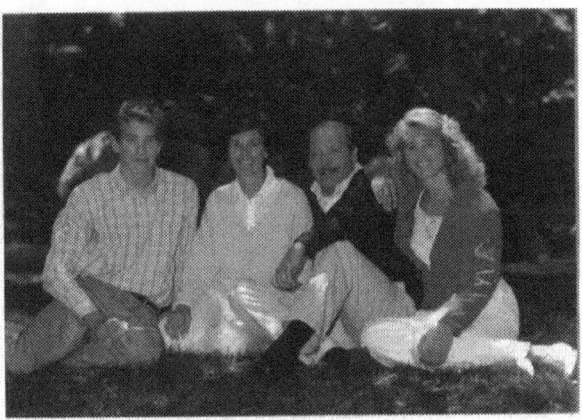

This picture is a little old. That is Adam on the far left, the beautiful Cathy, my ugly brother, the most beautiful Shay Lyn.

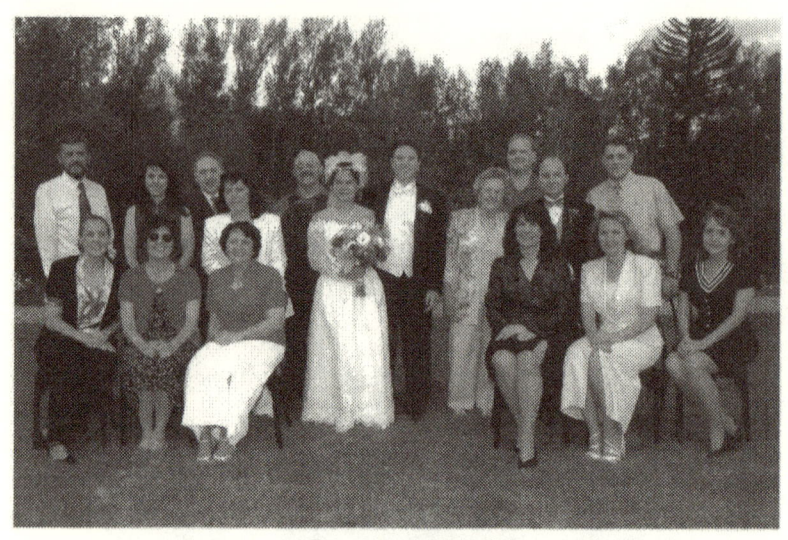

The Groeger family
top row left to right: Al, Lorie, Gene, Dennis, Dick, Thom.
Middle row: Lynne, Bob's youngest daughter Jackie Jean, the bride,
Elijah the groom,
Mom, Bob
front row: my Kathleen, Beth, Marcia, Donna, Cindy, Karen.

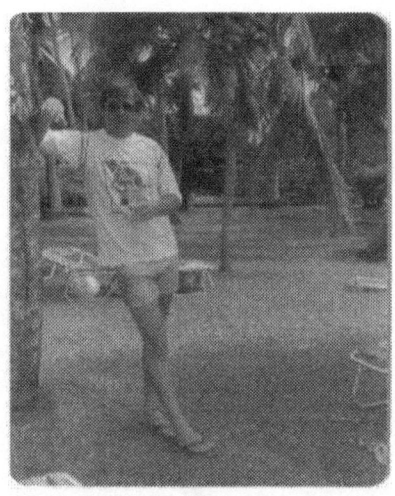

Beautiful, Beautiful Barbados. I am holding up a palm tree and drinking beer. What a great vacation. One I will never forget. Thanks Mom!

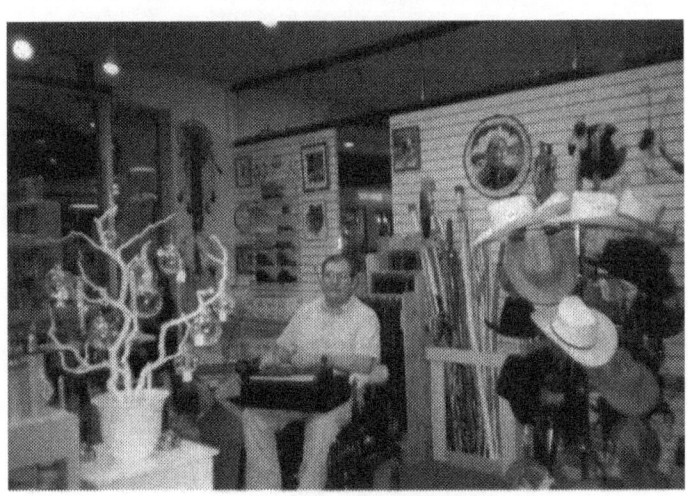

Me and my gift shop in Chapel Hills Mall

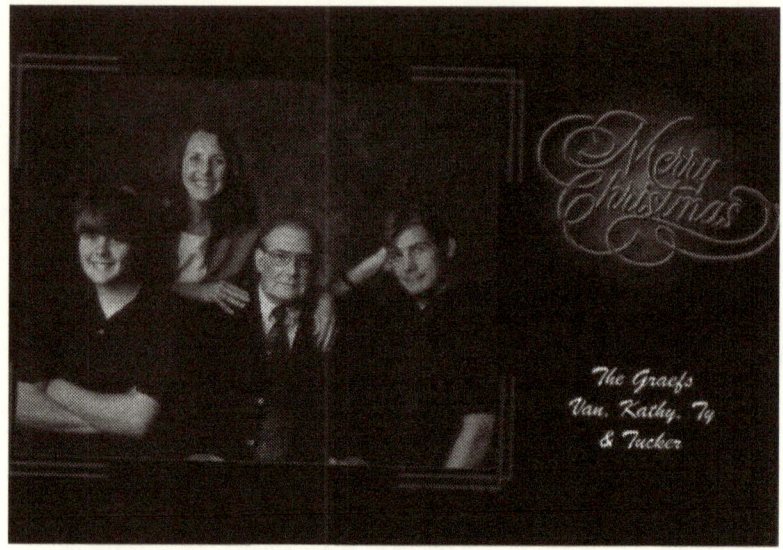

The Graefs
Van, Kathy, Ty
& Tucker

Two weeks before we lost Tucker, Kathleen decided that we should
have a family picture taken because I had been so sick. Little did we
know that we would lose Tucker.
Thanks to the greatest neighbors, Michale and Joyce for purchasing
these pictures for us.
These pictures were taken by:
LJM Photography Inc.
4642 North Park Drive
Colorado Springs, Colorado 80918
These folks are very professional and did a great job during our
tragedy.

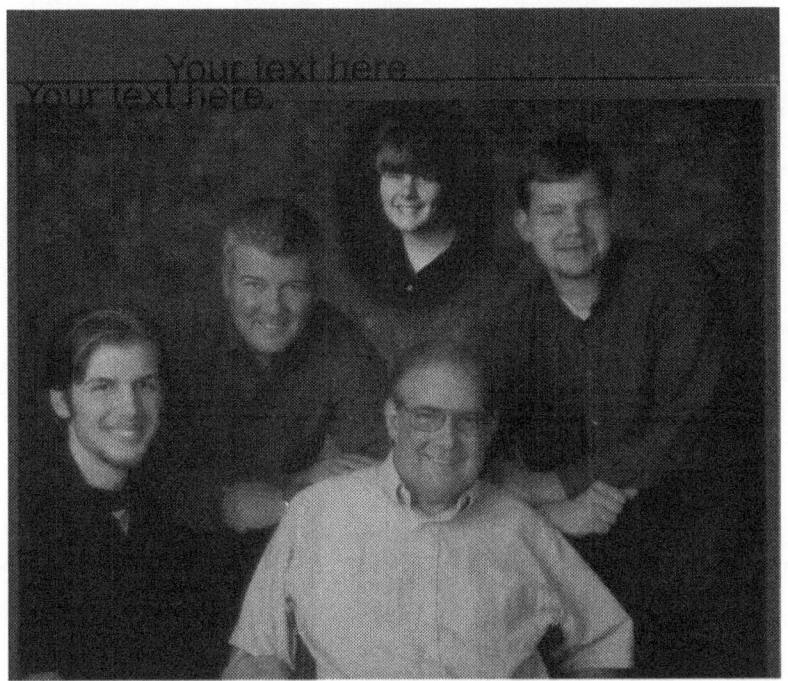

2 months after we lost Tucker, Kane and Mark came to see us and we had this picture taken and the photographer put Tucker in the picture. This is the last picture of my 4 boys ever

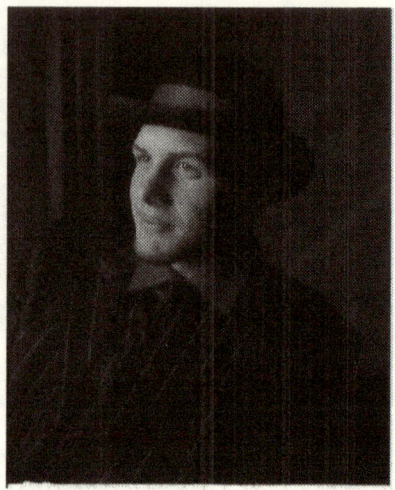

Number three son, Ty. What a gifted person in multiple areas. He really stepped forward on Tucker's catastrophe. He helped us to stay together at a real bad time. He graduates from Liberty High School in May of 2006. He is going to attend Colorado State University and will be studying in the medical field. Kathleen and I could not be more proud of our boy. Ty, nice hat.

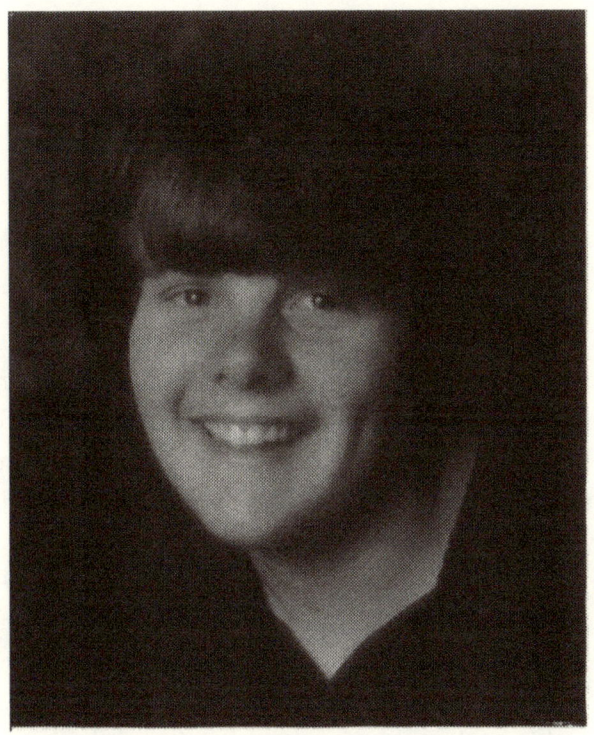

Our youngest son, Tucker, without whom this manuscript may
never have been written. We will always love him and will never
forget him
thanks son!

CHAPTER 10
Living with Kathleen

There we were in our new home, and I didn't have a job. I hadn't quit smoking, but Kathleen said that it was okay until I found a job. Before long, I landed a job with a company that leased automobiles to credit union members. The pay was good, but not great. Still, we could get by nicely with both our incomes.

I did quit smoking shortly after starting my job, and Dr. and Mrs. Groeger began to take me seriously. I always called Kathleen's dad "Doctor" out of respect. One day he told me that I was part of the family and I should call him Dad. Kathleen's family really took me in, and I felt like their fifteenth child. But then, I've heard the same thing from others who have been involved with the Groeger family. They had a way of making everyone feel like their fifteenth child.

Kathleen and I really enjoyed our new home. Kathleen was decorating and nesting, and I loved being able to go anywhere in the house. I had no obstacles to avoid. The bathroom was set up for a wheelchair, and I could get under the sink and transfer to the tall toilet. There was a ramp in the garage, and we later added ramps off the deck and front porch.

We were still doing a lot of fishing and traveled all over the state with our boat. I was still pretty mobile, and we developed quite a system for getting me into the boat. If there weren't any docks, Kathleen would transfer me from the wheelchair to the bow. I would hold onto whatever was available and shuffle myself to the right rear seat. If there was a dock, Kathleen would climb into the boat, slide me out of my chair on the dock, and pivot me to the seat in the stern.

We caught some great fish, and usually we would stop at Kathleen's parents' house on our way home to share what we had caught. They especially enjoyed the fresh trout.

Kathleen and I fished some beautiful spots in Colorado. There was a new reservoir west of Woodland Park, in a place called South Park. No kidding! South Park was located just west of the summit of Wilkerson Pass. The new reservoir was named Spiney Mountain, and it was just upstream from Eleven Mile Reservoir, which we fished often. These reservoirs were all on of the south branch of the Platte River.

The ride up Wilkerson Pass was a gradual incline, and we passed a lot of pine trees and aspen groves. When we got to the summit, it was beautiful. From the summit, we could look out over a flat stretch of land, then the lakes, and finally the Collegiate mountain range in the distance.

Before Spiney Mountain was open for fishing, it was stocked with rainbow and brown trout. They also tried something new, and stocked the reservoir with Snake River cutthroat trout. No one was able to fish the reservoir for several years.

When they finally opened it to fishing, Kathleen and I went to Spiney Mountain often. We could only fish with artificial bait, but one day I hooked a large fish. I asked Kathleen to net it for me, and tried to steer the fish towards us. I really wanted to watch Kathleen net that fish. It was a large cutthroat, about seven pounds. Kathleen and I just sat there with our mouths open when the fish took off toward the propeller and cut the line. How disappointing to have a big fish and lose it.

We made a pledge to each other that we would come back and get that big fish. We fished the reservoir several more times, with no luck. We did catch our share of nice-size trout, but the big one was playing hard to get.

One Saturday, we were on the water at sunrise, then fished all morning without any luck. It was almost noon when Kathleen and I agreed to go in and have lunch. I decided to troll a black Panther Martin on the way in to shore. As we turned toward the dock, I had a big strike on the lure. The fight was on. I knew whatever I had hooked was large. The fish was angry and really giving me a tussle. I was using a medium action spinning outfit with six-pound test line and was confident I had the right equipment to handle this fish. During the fight, a lot of things went through my mind. Did I tie the lure on securely, or was I in a hurry? I hope the fish won't get snagged on anything. Please don't let the line get cut on the propeller. I don't know how long I fought that fish, but it seemed like forever. My arms were really tired.

Finally, it was time for Kathleen to net the fish. I wasn't going to make the same mistake again. She could net the fish anywhere. Fortunately, it was all happening in front of me. I shouted to Kathleen to net her, and she did a beautiful job. We had a large, fat female cutthroat trout flopping in the bottom of the boat. Her colors were stunning, reds and pinks, with black speckles. The two red slashes under her chin were beautiful. She was six pounds and twenty-three inches long, and now hangs on our wall at home.

On one of our trips to Spiney Mountain, I hooked another large fish. When it came time to net the fish, Kathleen refused, saying, "I will not bring that ugly fish into this boat." The fish in question was a large northern pike. It looked like an alligator, and Kathleen wanted no part of it. We held it over the side of the boat, removed the hooks, and released it.

There is another reservoir on the western slope where we like to fish. It's five hours away from the Springs, but worth the trip. The Blue Mesa Reservoir is one of the largest in the state. It is the result of damming along the Gunnison River, and the fishing's not bad. Blue Mesa is just west of the little town of Gunnison, which is the home of Western State College, a nice liberal arts school. Crested Butte, a ski resort, is just north of town. Kathleen and I have talked about retiring in Gunnison. It's that type of mountain town.

The reservoir is surrounded by tall sandstone buttes. There aren't many trees, but there are a lot of tumbleweeds. Elk Creek Marina is about mid-lake, along with Pappy's Restaurant. The National Park begins just up from the marina and has facilities for campers, motor homes, and trailers. Elk Creek Marina opens onto a beautiful canyon, which registers over one hundred feet deep in some places on a depth finder.

During one of our trips to Blue Mesa Reservoir, I caught a Kokanee salmon. These are landlocked sock-eyed salmon that live in most of the high mountain lakes in Colorado. They only live for three to four years, then they turn red, spawn, and die. Every year after the fish have spawned, people try to snag the dying salmon, which just doesn't seem right to me.

The fish I had on my hook was just starting to turn red. He was only seventeen inches long, but he was pinkish, and his jaw was changing. These fish not only turn red, but they develop large, hooked jaws. This one was very unusual, so we had him mounted.

Kathleen and I did more than just fish. We had full-time jobs and entertained Kathleen's family a lot. I really enjoyed spending time with her brothers, sisters and parents. Because our house was wheelchair-accessible, it was just easier to have people come to our place.

◆   ◆   ◆

One year and a day after the wedding, our first son was born. We'd been warned that with multiple sclerosis, the reproductive function, if not the desire, is usually the first thing to go. Fortunately, it wasn't in my case. Kathleen went through the labor and delivery like she'd been doing it all her life. This time, I was in the room with her during the birthing process.

Kathleen had let me choose the baby's name, so I picked Kelly for a girl, and Ty for a boy. We named our first son Ty, after the famous baseball player Ty Cobb. I was still with the auto leasing company, and things were going well.

Three years passed, and my condition remained basically the same, with only a little physical deterioration. I didn't notice the little losses until they interrupted my normal lifestyle. My job was about to end, because the man who had started the business got sticky fingers and embezzled large sums of money. I was out of work again.

A friend, Gary, came to Chip and me with an idea for a business involving automobile financing for people with major credit problems. He had several financing sources who would handle customers with bad credit, and Chip and I had the knowledge and expertise to handle the automobile financing.

We really thought it was a great idea, and we each agreed to put in ten thousand dollars to get it started. Chip lent me ten thousand dollars so I could be involved in the project, and he also put in his own money. The three of us set out to make the idea go.

As secretary/treasurer, it was my job to do the documentation and all the computer work for the loans. We called the company Auto U.S./Colorado Springs, but had to become a used car dealership in order to buy the cars we needed. We bought cars at wholesale, sold them at retail, and collected a fee for doing the loan documentation. Selling warranties added a few bucks to the bottom line. We started out slowly, but grew quickly. There was a definite need for our services.

During this time, Kathleen and I added to our family. On October 10, 1990, our second son was born. Tucker was a little premature, but healthy. His name, of course, was my idea. People said he would get teased with a name like that, but I said, "He may get teased once, but that'll be all." With a name like Tucker, he needed to be strong and tough. And he was.

Kathleen originally wanted six children, but I'd bargained her down to three. We ended up with two, and we were done. I wasn't getting any younger.

The business did pretty well the first year. At one point, we employed nearly thirty people. We generated over a million dollars in gross sales. But given the cost of automobiles, we didn't see much profit. I think I took one $800 paycheck home. Chip and Gary took a little more. We moved the business to an obscure location, then hit a month where we didn't sell anything. That was our downfall. One night we disassembled the office and flew the coop. Gary, the president, took everything that wasn't nailed down. We didn't have much money, but it was gone, too.

I was left to handle all the garbage after we closed. We owed the government some money. Chip and I decided it would be better if we went to them before they came to us. We did, and we paid what we owed. The president got off scot-free because he was gone, and the government didn't care if he owned sixty percent of the company when my brother and I were standing right there in front of them.

I had to deal with all kinds of company-related things for nearly a year before it was finally over. Then I had to pay Chip back the money he lent me.

The one thing I learned from that business was that I really preferred working for myself. With the possibility of my health getting worse, I could work at my own pace without the threat of being fired. I decided that if I was going to work, it would only be for myself.

So there I was with a wife, two children, and no job once again. During this time, Kane and Mark would come to Colorado every year for at least two weeks. If they could, they would stay longer with us, and we would go fishing, camping, and stuff like that. Kathleen truly loved my boys and treated them like they were her own.

After the business failed, I had to sell my boat. It was a great little fishing boat, but I had no trouble selling it, since we needed to eat. Physically, I was still doing about the same. I wasn't walking much, but I was still standing with the help of a dresser or Kathleen. I could still write and do most things with my right hand.

◆   ◆   ◆

On December 7, 1990, Kathleen's dad passed away. He had been fighting cancer, and hadn't been feeling well for a year or two. We all took his passing very hard, and we still miss him today.

◆   ◆   ◆

One day, I was sitting at home watching TV when a Kathleen's sister's friend, Lynne, came by to talk to me. Denis Green had a ranch up in the mountains and was known as the Mystery Man of the Mountains. He manufactured brass jewelry and asked me if I was interested in selling it.

Denis said he would give me some jewelry on consignment. He told me to just go out and show it, and people would buy it. I had a little trouble believing it was that easy, but I tried it. When I showed it, people did buy it, and selling it was fun. I took the jewelry to craft fairs just before Christmas and did pretty well. I told Denis that our family had the best Christmas ever because of his jewelry.

After Christmas, there were no craft shows, and people just weren't buying. I decided I needed a new audience. Carrying all the jewelry around was getting difficult, so I went to the local mall, Citadel, to set up a cart to sell the jewelry. When I asked Denis if he would consign additional jewelry to me so that I could fill up the cart, he said he would, and we were off and running.

Even during the slow part of the retail year, we still did okay. Laurel Harris, a friend of mine, helped me, and we worked the cart for ten weeks.

Laurel was an attractive Christian girl who wanted to be an actress. She had even gone to Hollywood once, and had gotten a few roles as an extra. She had come home and was doing some TV work with the Methodist Church. I always told her that she would make it someday.

Just the other day, I saw her in a national commercial on the History Channel on cable television. She also sent us a Christmas card, saying that she had just finished filming an independent movie, but I never heard any more about that. When Laurel quit the store, we were involved in a disagreement over something in our original agreement.

It was not easy doing business from a cart in the mall. Just about the time customers started to remember our location, the mall management would move our cart. I thought it was a good time to expand, so I went to Chapel Hills Mall to arrange for another cart. Chapel Hills was newer and was located three miles west of my house. The management was looking for people to open stores, so they offered me a store for the same cost as a cart. I thought that would be a good deal, and I had met several people at the first mall who said they would consign their products to me if I opened a store.

We closed the cart and focused on opening the store. With Denis Green's jewelry, some leather goods, and some southwestern pots, we opened the store. We called it Colorado Reflections. Except for Laurel's wages, all the money went back into the store for new inventory. We tried to limit the store to Colorado-made souvenirs and products, but, over time, that became more and more difficult to do. Most souvenirs were made in Taiwan or China, but we ran with what we had.

My condition stayed about the same, except that I experienced more fatigue and had less endurance. When Kathleen saw me fighting to climb the ramp to get into the house, she decided it was time for a power wheelchair. I adapted quickly to pushing a joystick rather than the wheels of my chair. My first power chair was an Invacare XT, and it really was a neat chair. It had small knobby balloon tires, all the same size. The chair looked like a little tank. It was very powerful, and good for outdoor traveling.

I was still doing some fly fishing with Chip. The new chair really helped me get down to the streams. We liked to fish the South Platte River. There's a section between Spiney Mountain Reservoir and Eleven Mile Reservoir that is designated a gold medal trout stream. It was fly fishing only, lure only, and catch and release. This section of stream ran through a treeless meadow between the two reservoirs. I could still cast the fly line pretty well. One day I got a little adventurous and tried to move downstream a bit. All of a sudden my right front wheel went into a ground squirrel hole, and I couldn't get it out. I'd still be there if it weren't for some nice fishermen. I learned I couldn't go everywhere.

Our next trip out, my brother helped me set up on a bend of the stream, near a large pool. I was situated just below the pool, before the fast water. Right in front of me lay a large rainbow trout, feeding. I thought to myself, <u>This is going to be easy.</u> It wasn't easy. This fish could tell the difference between real and fake. Every fisherman that passed by had to stop and cast for him. The wise old trout would consider their offer, but wouldn't strike.

I had matched the hatch and was using exactly what the fish was feeding on. But then, everyone was using the same fly. Mine was tied to a number twenty hook. This particular stream is known for having large hatches of these little green bugs. After sitting there for about two hours, I noticed that when the fish approached my offering, it would take a long glance before turning away. I knew I was destined to catch this big rainbow. Then I realized that the fish could see where the leader met the fly line. With a short cast, I lifted the fly line out of the water, and left the leader and fly in the water.

It worked, and the big fish sucked in my little fly. I set the hook and raised the tip of my rod. The fish took off up stream. All I could do was to hold my hand over my reel and hang on. The trout made some very acrobatic leaps to rid itself of my hook. After a lot of give and take, the fish was mine.

Now my major problem was that I couldn't reach the fish to unhook it. A nice couple came by, saying, "You finally got that booger." They offered to help me remove the hook and to measure the fish for me.

The fish was twenty-five inches long, and approximately five pounds. The couple who helped me were real nice, but in removing the fly, they bent my hook so badly it couldn't be used. It was the last fly I had of its type, and there were a lot more fish in the pool to catch. About then, Chip showed up. He wasn't having much luck, so we decided to just go home.

◆   ◆   ◆

I was not yet forty-five years old on January 12, 1994, when I woke up at 3:32 a.m. with what I thought was bad heartburn. Kathleen called 911. First came the firemen, walking through the house with their boots on. Then came the paramedics who, like Kathleen, thought I was having a heart attack. My chest hurt, but it wasn't that bad. I wasn't scared, and I had no sense of impending death. Just to be safe, they rushed me out of the house and into an ambulance.

I thought it was funny that they asked me the best way to get to the hospital. Maybe they were testing me to see how alert I was. The paramedics gave me a nitroglycerin tablet to put under my tongue, to see if it relieved the pain, but I don't recall that it did anything. They kept asking me how bad the pain was, on a scale of one to ten. I told them if a kidney stone was a ten, this was a seven or eight.

At the hospital, the doctors confirmed I was having a heart attack. They finally gave me some pain medication that helped, and then sent me to the coronary care unit. I have always told Kathleen that I didn't want drastic measures taken to keep me alive, and she stayed with me the whole time. After the pain medication kicked in, I fell asleep. When I woke up, they asked me if I still had pain. At first I didn't, but then it came back and they gave me more pain medication. It was good stuff, that Demerol. I couldn't take morphine because it had made me violently ill during a kidney stone episode.

The cardiologist decided we'd better take a look inside and scheduled a procedure, using dye, that would show any blockages in my arteries. Kathleen and I both warned him not to go in through my legs because of my spasticity, but no one paid attention to us. In the middle of the procedure, I felt a spasm, and saw a very concerned look on the doctor's face. Afraid he had dissected my artery, he said, "I better get out now." I spent the night in the intensive care unit, and they checked me every hour to make sure I wasn't bleeding internally. A few days later, the doctors decided to go back in through my arm, as we had suggested in the beginning.

I had one artery that was ninety percent blocked. They waited a couple of days, then did an angioplasty through my other arm to clear the blockage. Everything went fine, and I didn't have to have open heart surgery. After the heart attack, my multiple sclerosis really flared up. I lost use of my left hand almost completely, and my right hand didn't work that well, either. I was so tired, I couldn't do the work at the store without help. Kathleen thought that I needed a new wheelchair that reclined, so I got an Invacare XT with a recliner system. Within a week or two, I was back at the store selling souvenirs.

Laurel had quit by this time, and I hired the little girl who had been working at the GNC store. Diana Dawn Ridley was another cute little blonde, and everyone called her Dee Dee. She enjoyed country western dancing, and when Kane came to visit, I thought they might hit it off, but it wasn't meant to be. Dee Dee married a cadet from the Air Force Academy, and they have two beautiful children. They move quite often, but Dee Dee calls me every once in a while.

The store was fun to operate, and we were paying all the bills. I still wasn't taking a paycheck for myself. The mall management considered us a temporary tenant. We were on a month-to-month lease, so at any given time, if a permanent tenant wanted our space, we would have to leave. We were very fortunate for the first three years, but I began to think it might be a good idea to lease a permanent location in the mall. The store was paying for itself, and it looked like something I would be able to handle for a while. I negotiated a five-year lease on a location not far from the old spot, except that it was upstairs. Still, it was near the food court.

After we moved the store upstairs, it started off slow. And it stayed slow, no matter what kind of advertising we did. Nothing seemed to help, not even the television commercial we had done.

CHAPTER 11
Dream or Nightmare?
Mickey Finn's

One night I was talking to Kathleen's older sister, Lynne, about what we really wanted to do with our lives. She was a physician's assistant but didn't think she wanted to do that forever. I didn't want to run the store for the rest of my life, either. She said, "Wouldn't it be nice to own our own sports bar?"

It was a great idea. I could picture myself owning a sports bar. After all, I had frequented my share of bars. And what would be a more natural setting for me than a sports bar? I had some bartending experience, and enough banking knowledge to handle the finances. It was worth looking into.

We agreed I would do the research to see what the possibilities were. I started looking through entrepreneur magazines and found a franchise that sounded pretty good. It was a small company, so the franchise fee wasn't too steep. The investment would be nothing like opening a McDonald's. Their franchise company had eight or nine locations, and they were headquartered in Omaha, Nebraska. I called and requested their brochure, then showed it to Lynne, who thought it looked pretty good. When I showed it to some friends at the mall, we all agreed there wasn't anything like that at or near the mall. Everyone I spoke to liked the idea of having somewhere to stop after a long day's work. I approached the assistant manager of the mall. He thought it was a great idea, and he thought the mall would be very interested.

Lynne suggested we talk to the franchise people and see what they had to offer. I called and made an appointment for them to meet us at the mall. Our initial meeting went well, and we found out how much money we would need to get started. We'd found a location at the mall that was formerly a deli, and the mall management said they would help us renovate the space. Things were going along just fine.

In the midst of all this negotiating, I realized Colorado Reflections was not doing well. I had shifted my focus from my store to the sports bar. The staff I had hired to keep Colorado Reflections going just wasn't doing its job. I realized I'd better make a choice and concentrate on either the store or the sports bar.

I decided to close the store and focus on starting the sports bar. The first obstacle I had to overcome was my five-year lease with the mall. I turned to a local attorney, Pete Lee, for help. Pete had helped a couple of Kathleen's brothers and sisters. He got me out of the lease, and I closed Colorado Reflections. When I asked, Pete said he could also help me with the paperwork to purchase the sports bar.

By this time, Lynne was having second thoughts. She didn't have any money to live on if she quit her job to help run the business, and she didn't want to risk her house. I asked several people who I thought would be interested in doing this type of a deal. At first, everyone was interested, but when it came to discussing money, they all backpedaled pretty quickly.

Kathleen and I decided to find a way to do it on our own. The first chore was to find a location. My first choice was the mall, and the franchise agreed. They already had one bar in a mall, and it was doing well. We made an appointment with the upper management at the mall, thinking we had a good deal going in. Ten minutes into the meeting, we got blown out. The mall felt we would be too small to handle the traffic they were planning. They were going to add an ice rink and do some other remodeling, and a small, local sports bar just wasn't in their plans. A Ruby Tuesday's eventually went into the spot we wanted.

Any change in location had to be approved by the franchise. I had a friend in real estate who said she would help us. The franchise had looked around and made some suggestions about location. Their new first choice wasn't available, either. We looked and looked, but didn't find anything we, or the franchise, liked. One day, my realtor friend called to say the second location the franchise approved had become available.

The location was a mile from my house and two miles from the mall. The franchise liked it because of all the "rooftops" in the area. We contacted the owner and started negotiations. Pete Lee had helped us set up a company called Extra Innings, LLC, and Kathleen and I were the officers. The franchise was really interested in us now. They said if we prepaid a portion of the franchise fee, they would help us negotiate with the property owner. Kathleen and I coughed up the fee, and negotiations really got going. The franchise people were really knowledgeable, and we felt we had gotten a pretty good deal.

Now Kathleen and I had to come up with the financing. Our credit was in great shape, and I thought it would be a quick thing to get done. I applied everywhere, but no one was interested in financing a bar. I finally hired an agency with sources that would do this type of lending.

By now, several months had gone by, and we still didn't have our loan. Lou Christiansen, the owner of the location, was getting upset. We liked him, and he liked us, so he agreed to work with us. Kathleen and I tried to decide what we should do, and she suggested that a couple of her siblings might be interested in helping us out.

After a couple more months, we finally made a deal with her brother, Thom, and her brother-in-law, Brad. We had the front money we needed, but not the money for remodeling the store. The current location had been in business for ten years as a place called Good Company. Kathleen and I had often taken the boys there to eat in the past, but once the current owner bought it and let his son run the place, it had really gone downhill. The last time Kathleen and I had eaten there, we'd decided we would never go back. The food wasn't very good, and the place was dirty. It would need a complete overhaul to make it work.

The franchise got involved again and made a deal with Mr. Christiansen to take back a loan for the remodeling. Believe it or not, we had a date to close on the business. Now we had to get a liquor license from the city. Thank God for Pete Lee. He handled the whole thing, which was not easy. Our closing date was May 16, 1997, but there were inspections required, along with a final approval on our liquor license. The franchise people were sitting at our dining room table at 8:00 a.m. on the 16th of May, waiting for the final word on our liquor license. At 9:00 a.m., we finally got the okay and prepared to go to the closing at 10:00 a.m.

After all the negotiations, the financing was in place, but Kathleen got a little nervous. She didn't want to lose the house. I explained that the absolute worst thing that could happen would be that we'd have to declare bankruptcy if the business didn't work out. But I was very confident that it would work, and the franchise had assured us it would. It had been a long time since we'd toyed with the original idea. Along the way, we decided more than once that it was never going to happen, and the franchise people had their doubts, too. Well, it was finally happening, and Kathleen and I owned a sports bar/restaurant. We decided to keep Good Company open and keep the current staff. We planned to do all the remodeling at night and on Sundays, when Good Company was closed.

I remember the very first night after we became the owners. I was sitting at a table and couldn't believe that the place was ours. Kathleen wasn't there, but my friend, Ron, was helping me celebrate. What did he care? He was drinking for free. As I looked around the bar, I saw a lot of Good Company's regular customers. The bar had gotten a bad reputation in the past five years, and there were some pretty suspicious characters hanging around. We would definitely change the clientele when we changed the name to Mickey Finn's.

We had enough cash to do all the remodeling. One of the franchise group, John Vones, stayed with us to help turn Good Company into Mickey Finn's. We kept the place open six days a week, and we were making money while we remodeled. We put in new carpet and new wallpaper, painted the ceilings, and wainscoted the whole store. Chip was selling signs at the time, and we ordered signs for both the front and the back of the building.

One of my projects was to decorate the inside with sports pictures. After all, Colorado Springs was the amateur sports center of the country. The city boasts the Olympic Training Center, two local colleges, a ton of softball teams, and the Sky Sox, the Rockies AAA team. In Denver, you could find the Broncos, the Rockies, and the Avalanche, not to mention the downtrodden Nuggets.

A photographer next door to the bar helped me with a few pictures, and a local lady helped me frame two Bronco jerseys. Chip had gone to a flea market somewhere and bought me a whole bunch of old-time baseball pictures of Mickey Mantle, Don Drysdale, and a lot of the famous Yankees and Dodgers. We had installed seven brand new twenty-seven inch televisions. We also had a projection screen, which was five feet square. We set up a dart area with plastic darts and an electronic game board, had a video golf game put in, and bought a pinball machine. We'd left room for a Foosball table.

I bought an automatic door opener to turn the front door into a handicapped entrance. The bathrooms were in decent shape, but the kitchen needed a little work. There was a nice patio outside the back door, and it overlooked Pike's Peak.

The patio was above the road level, and the tables all had umbrellas. Kathleen noticed that the kitchen help had been making themselves at home in the back, where they smoked and took their breaks. It wasn't a very pretty sight from the patio tables. My Kathleen went out and bought wood and cement. She built a beautiful wooden fence, so that the people on the patio would not see the kitchen help smoking. John, the guy from the franchise group, helped us all he could to understand what had to be done.

I selected a girl who'd worked for Good Company to be the new manager. We were really gearing up for the grand opening. We had done a mailing in the neighborhood to attract the locals. Mickey Finn's sure was looking nice.

On our grand opening day, everyone showed up. Kathleen's brothers and sisters came, along with people from the hospital, friends of ours, Pete Lee, and all the folks from the franchise group. There were also a bunch of other people we finally decided were customers.

John from the franchise hung around for a couple more weeks. Kathleen and I both thought he did a great job. One of the reasons I'd wanted to go the franchise route was that we didn't have the expertise to run a bar and restaurant, and we were willing to pay them to teach us.

Being in a wheelchair put me at a disadvantage because there were some places I couldn't get into, such as the bathrooms, the kitchen, and the area behind the bar. I could get into the office, but then the door wouldn't close. I would sit out by the bar, watching people to make sure that things were going okay. I met a lot of our customers. The staff that worked for us in the beginning had all worked at the old place. Not all of them had great reputations.

The second night Mickey Finn's was open, one of the bartenders came in drunk, and he continued to get worse as the night went on. I watched him and saw that each time he made a drink for a customer, he would take a gulp for himself. By 9:00 p.m., he couldn't work the cash register, so we told him that somebody would take over his shift. He went around the bar and told everyone we had fired him, then left with about five customers, which was okay, because they hadn't been paying for their drinks anyway.

During the next couple of weeks, we noticed a lot of things missing, such as beer, corned beef, liquor, and money. The sad thing was, if any one of our employees had needed any of the things they stole, we would have been more than happy to give it to them. I must have been an easy mark. When we finally let a second bartender go, we increased our nightly take by several hundred dollars. This guy had been working five nights a week and was my friend to my face.

The biggest problem I had as a manager was that I could not stay late. Our investors, my brothers-in-law, had both asked me how I was going to manage the bar if I wasn't there. I told them we would hire good managers, and I truly believed it at the time, but that is much easier said than done. We gradually replaced most of the people who had worked for the old store, but the new people were not that great, either.

In January, 1998, the franchise was having a convention in Las Vegas. Kathleen and I could not afford to go, and said so. They said they really wanted us there and would pay for our hotel room. We took advances from our credit cards, and we headed for Las Vegas with the kids. It took us two long days to drive it, but we finally got there, and we enjoyed meeting some of the other franchisees. Then it came to our meeting with the franchise people. I'd always thought that a convention was supposed be fun, but these people seemed to be there just to beat me up. A disgruntled employee we'd fired had called the franchise group and told them that our employees and managers were selling drugs at the bar. The franchise told us to get rid of our manager, or they would force us to close our doors. To say the least, it was a terrible weekend, and I had no desire to go back to Las Vegas. Kathleen and the kids really enjoyed themselves, but when the kids ask when we're going back to Las Vegas, the answer is, "Never."

Our manager, Jaime, had just offered to lend us twenty-five thousand dollars to help keep the business afloat. Now we couldn't take her money, and we had to fire her. Suddenly, John was hanging around the bar, apparently representing the franchise group. She never had gotten along with him, so she made herself scarce. I really liked Jaime. She had been diagnosed with multiple sclerosis, too, and was handling it quite well. She was a Native American, whose Cherokee grandfather had taught her a lot of American Indian ways. She made one drink from hundred-year-old mushrooms. She'd been making me this concoction on a daily basis, and, believe it or not, it really helped my hands. So now we had lost out on her friendship, her investment, and her medical knowledge.

The franchise made me hire a guy with a lot of restaurant and bar experience. His salary was more than we could afford, but after a few weeks, he came to me and suggested that we get rid of the franchise group. He said we could change the name of the place, and he'd help get the new place going.

Somehow, it seemed easier for me to deal with all my work-related problems if I had a few cocktails before Kathleen picked me up at the end of the day. One evening after Kathleen drove me home, we got into a huge fight, and I decided to take myself back to the bar in my chair. It was 7:00 and already dark outside, and Kathleen didn't think that was such a great idea. I had gotten halfway up the block when she caught up to me and, without saying a word, turned the power off on my chair. Then she took it out of gear by flipping levers at the bottom of the chair, in a place I couldn't reach. I could not move.

She pushed me back to the house and proceeded to put me to bed against my will. I had absolutely no control over the situation, and I was devastated to realize that I could be put in such a predicament.

We have talked about this episode many times. I think I know why she did what she did, and I think she knows how I felt, too. Fortunately, we have never gotten to that point again, and we both pray it never happens.

◆   ◆   ◆

I called Pete Lee to help us get rid of the franchise. I expected it to be difficult, but he certainly handled the whole thing easily. I hoped that without paying that five percent franchise fee per week, we'd show a profit. We started out by changing the menu, then the hours of operation, and then finally the name of the restaurant. I made the mistake of asking for customer input, offering a prize for the best new name. Everyone but the leasing lady got upset because their favorite name wasn't chosen.

Changing a restaurant's menus and a bar's liquor license are major undertakings. Right in the midst of the transition, the guy who was going to lead us out of our franchise quit. We had a mess on our hands, but one of the managers and I did our best to get the new place going. Menus and signs aren't cheap, but the Rampart Inn was about to open.

It was now November, 1998, and we were late with the rent. When I went to the leasing people to see if they could help us, they said there just wasn't anything they could do. Kathleen and I had a long, serious conversation about what we should do. The place had really been a drag on our relationship, and I told her I'd rather have her than any dumb old bar and restaurant.

It was Monday or Tuesday of the week, and we planned to close the restaurant down for good on Sunday. On Wednesday, one of my employees and her husband came to me and asked if we would sell the place to them. We made a deal and kept the Rampart Inn open, and they started all the necessary work to buy it.

In order for us to buy the place originally, Kathleen and I had put all our money into it. We did sell it for more than we paid for it, but we had also spent a lot of money on the renovations. In order to break even, we would have had to sell the place for twice the amount we paid. Still, just getting it off our hands was a relief, and Bruce and Trish were nice people. They had been customers of Good Company and wanted to change the place back. And that's just what they did. As far as I know, they still own it today.

When Kathleen and I had put everything we had into this deal, we expected to have enough income that Kathleen could work part-time at the hospital and spend more time with the kids. After owning the place for a year and a half, I'd been there every day and never taken out a dime. After all was said and done, Kathleen and I had accumulated a lot of debt. When we sold the bar, a major portion of the debt was paid off, but we still owed a whole lot of money, and we had no choice but to take legal action to protect ourselves.

After the sale of the bar, I pretty much stayed at home, doing a lot of follow-up work on closing Extra Innings, LLC. Altogether, between the state and federal requirements, that took well over a year.

◆   ◆   ◆

Just prior to closing the bar, I'd had the pleasure of spending time with my mother, who was suffering from emphysema. We spent the day talking, and it was a nice visit. The following day, we got a call from Chip, who said he needed help cleaning her up after she'd had a B.M. Kathleen talked to him, then suggested he call 911 because Mom wasn't responding appropriately.

The EMTs had to intubate her at the scene. She was taken to the hospital and put on a ventilator. In a short time, we had all gathered at the hospital. The doctor told us that Mom had suffered an internal bleed and was not responsive. My mother had told me that she did not want to continue to live the way she was living. She had breathing problems and was very limited in her activities. She would spend all day and night in her recliner, because she couldn't breathe when she lay down flat. She had been in her recliner when Chip discovered her. She had a living will that clearly stated that she did not want heroic measures, including intubation, taken to keep her alive. The doctors said if she stayed on the ventilator, more than likely she would be in a vegetative state. Chip and I made the decision to honor her wishes. In accordance with her living will, we asked to have the ventilator removed, and within a short time, she passed away.

Our father passed away almost a year to the day after our mother. He died in a Florida nursing home, and the people down there took care of everything. My father was eighty-four years old at the time of his death, and I know he never expected to live that long, because he told me once that he was having financial difficulties because he hadn't planned that far in advance. I couldn't go to Florida, and Chip refused to go. My brother and I were now orphans.

CHAPTER 12
Seeing the Light

Kathleen has always looked out for my well-being, so if I develop a problem, we have it checked out. When I began to have a lot of bladder infections, we went to a urologist. He suggested doing an ultrasound of my bladder to see if I was voiding completely. Sure enough, I had a stone in my bladder the size of a golf ball.

The doctor explained that there was a procedure that would explode the stone. It was an outpatient procedure, but, fortunately, they did knock me out, because they had to insert an instrument up through my penis to reach the stone. Afterward, the doctor said all went well.

When I turned fifty, the neurologist, Toni McClellan, suggested I have both ends scoped and my prostate checked. They put a scope down my throat to make sure that my heartburn had not caused any damage. The procedure at the other end, of course, was to check for polyps and cancer. They knock you out for these, too. Then they blow air up your butt to expand your intestine so the scope will fit inside. They only went up through my small intestine. If you're fortunate enough to wake up during the procedure, as I did, you can see your own poop chute.

Afterward, they put you in a recovery room with a bunch of other people who have had the same procedure. You can imagine what happens next. All that air has to be expelled sooner or later, and the place was like a frat house. Kathleen and I thought we would never stop laughing.

◆   ◆   ◆

I get the local multiple sclerosis newsletter. One day there was an article in it about a new procedure, written by my neurologist. When we contacted her, she didn't make any promises, but said it might help me. It was a chemo drug called Novantron, and the one stipulation was that you couldn't have any heart disease. I thought for sure I would be disqualified because of my heart attack, but I went in and had an ultrasound of my heart done. The cardiologist said I was fine, but suggested a change in my blood pressure medication. We went back to the neurologist to set up the new procedure. Like anything else, it had to be approved by the health insurance company, which could take some time.

At the neurologist's office, we discussed a lot of things besides the cancer drug. I was having trouble with my right hand, and we were concerned because my left hand was basically not functioning at all. We didn't want my right hand to get that way, so the neurologist suggested that I go on steroids to help my right hand. This would be an intravenous treatment that we could manage for a week at home. A nurse came to the house and set up the intravenous equipment. Of course, my Kathleen handled the procedure.

It had been a couple of weeks since my heart ultrasound. My old blood pressure medication, Lopressor, had been replaced with Zestril. The week of the Solu Medrol, the intravenous steroid, had ended on Saturday. That night, April 30, 2001, I had a slight sore throat, but didn't think much about it. Sunday morning I woke up pretty early and told Kathleen that I was having a little trouble swallowing. I asked her to help me up so I could have coffee. She just smiled, and I realized how silly my request sounded.

Kathleen went to the store and bought some cough drops and throat spray. We tried them, and they didn't work. The sore throat was getting worse, so much so that I really couldn't swallow without a lot of pain. After a few hours, Kathleen said, "We're going to the hospital." At first I resisted, but the pain kept getting worse, so I gave in and we went to the emergency room, leaving the boys by themselves.

We checked in and sat in the waiting room. By this time, the pain was really bad and my eyes had started to water, but I was still breathing pretty well through my nose. Kathleen went and talked to someone and told them that I was really in pain. When they finally took me back to a room, Dr. Watts came in and did a quick examination. He said, "As long as you're not having any trouble breathing, that's the main thing."

Kathleen, bless her soul, asked the doctor if I could have some pain medication. He said yes. Two young nurses must have stuck me ten times without finding a vein in my arm.

The doctor moved to the examining room next door, where a forty-year-old women thought she was having a heart attack. She had been out running when she got chest pains. She must've been pretty or something, because there were a lot of guys in there. Kathleen was a little upset that this woman was getting all the attention.

Suddenly, I started to have trouble breathing. That brought Dr. Watts back in a hurry. The first time he'd examined me, he had asked me to open my mouth so he could look at my throat. I hadn't been able to do it, and he hadn't pressed the issue. This time, he forced my mouth open, then yelled for a respiratory therapist. She appeared very quickly, what they call "stat." I recognized Kim, the therapist, and remember smiling at her. As the doctor yelled some instructions to her, I was gone.

I haven't talked about religion or God yet, but I will later. The experience that I had at that moment is a story in itself. I was in a place where there was a beautiful blue stream of light. Something told me to step into the stream, which I did. The stream was moving up toward a very bright light. I suddenly realized that I was standing and had no pain. This was a very calm place, and I knew exactly what to do without anyone telling me. I felt totally at peace, with no pain, no worries, and no multiple sclerosis.

As I looked at the light, there seemed to be a door, like a storm door. A person was waving to me from behind that door. As I got closer, I recognized the person as someone I had known as a kid. He was smiling and waving to me to come to him. We used to call him Uncle Henry, and he lived upstairs in the house that my mother, my brother, and I lived in when I was in high school. He was the landlady's brother and had retired from the railroad. Every month when his pension came in, he would go out and drink. We would find him in the street, or in the bushes next to the house. My mother would always bring him in and try to sober him up so his sister and her husband wouldn't get mad at him. He was really a nice old man, but I had not thought about him in at least thirty-five years.

I was still heading toward Uncle Henry, when I suddenly I woke up in the intensive care unit. Kathleen was very upset, and she told me that they had almost lost me. They'd cut open my throat so I could breathe. Good old Dr. Watts had saved my life. I couldn't talk because of the tube in my throat, which was pretty sore. Every so often, they would come in and suck junk out of my throat with a machine. I went back to sleep, and then woke up to find Kathleen's sister Lynne and my brother Chip sitting in the room. I couldn't talk, but I really wanted to tell them what I had experienced. I kept pointing to the light on the ceiling, hoping they would understand what I was trying to say. They didn't.

Kathleen told me what had gone on in the emergency room. The doctor had instructed Kim, the respiratory therapist, to get air into my lungs. She told him that air was going in, but wasn't coming out, and she was afraid that she was going to burst my lungs. Kathleen saw what was going on and asked the doctor if she should leave. Dr. Watts said yes, and Kathleen left the exam room.

My friend Kim told Kathleen that when the doctor had cut into my throat, blood flew all over the place. Once they got me breathing, Kim said they took me for a CAT scan of my throat. I don't remember it, but she said that I asked for Kathleen. Kim said that I turned very blue. Perhaps that was when I was in the blue stream.

The medical explanation was that I had had an allergic reaction to my new blood pressure medicine. I think what I had was a near-death experience. I couldn't wait to tell someone about it.

After going through such an experience, I thought for sure that my life should become special or charmed. It just felt as though something should change, but after a few days, I realized I was just the same asshole I had always been. Still, I had a burning desire to tell people about my experience. By the fourth day in intensive care, I was able to talk, so I immediately told Kathleen. She was very interested in what I had seen and wanted to know more. The people in the intensive care unit were great, and they really took care of Kathleen and me.

That whole episode really stressed Kathleen out. Her boss realized it and offered her some time off, which was great. She got to stay with me in the hospital and at home for nearly seven weeks. I really needed her with me, and she really needed the time off.

I couldn't wait to tell some of my Christian friends about my experience. I was very disappointed when they were not as excited as I was. They didn't take me seriously. When that happened more than once, I began to feel as though I probably shouldn't tell anyone else, so I stopped telling people the story.

Before that experience, I had never wanted to be resuscitated if something happened. I didn't want any special means used to keep me alive, and those had been my instructions to Kathleen. But now things were different. The next time Kathleen asked me about using heroic means, I told her to do whatever was necessary, and since then I've been glad I told her that. I feel there is a lot left for me to do here. I have my Kathleen and my boys, and maybe I can help someone else somehow.

One Sunday morning, I was watching a television show called <u>Angels, Miracles, and Afterlife</u>, about near-death experiences. Each person's experience was different. But then they started showing one person's experience, and I freaked. He'd seen exactly the same thing I had seen, except for who was standing at the door. Of course, there was no one with me at the time, so I couldn't show anyone what I saw. I tried to watch the show every Sunday, in case they played that episode again. I never saw it come back on, and then the station took the show off the air.

About a week after I got out of the hospital following the swollen throat incident, I started my chemo treatment. The timing wasn't great, but I was anxious to see if the chemo would help. I certainly wasn't excited about the possibility of losing my hair, but the neurologist said it was a small dose, and might not affect my follicles.

When I entered the big room where the chemo would take place, there were several patients already in the room getting their treatments. These people were sick. They were getting their chemo because they really needed it, and I felt guilty for being there. They gave me several medications to prevent stomach problems, which seemed to work, and then the chemo.

The pretreatment drugs made me feel a little better the first day. Then I was a mess for two weeks afterward, tired and weak, and I just didn't want to do anything. The neurologist said that patients were feeling better after two or three doses. I got a dose every three months. Originally, they said you could only receive a total of eight doses in your lifetime. Now they were recommending twelve doses in a lifetime. I did not want four more treatments. Enough was too much. But the neurologist told me that the Novantrone was keeping the multiple sclerosis at bay.

I was still having some UTIs, and the urologist thought I should have a KUB. They take an x-ray of your whole urinary tract, from your kidneys to your bladder. And so, of course, I had the X-ray done. I had several stones stuck in my kidney. The urologist suggested a new procedure that used sound waves to shatter the stones. It was another outpatient procedure, and they knocked me out, because if they didn't, lithotripsy would hurt. They used to perform the procedure underwater, but with this new technology, they didn't use the water anymore. After the procedure was complete, I went back and had another KUB done just to make sure all the stones were gone. They'd gotten all the stones except for one that was stuck in my urethra, and the doctor said that, with luck, I should pee it out later. I did.

PICTURES BY NAME ON PAGE 189. PICTURES GO ACROSS IN SOME WHAT CHRONOLOGICALLY ORDER.

voice activated p. 1 and 2,

Chip and me,

football picture,

All County baseball,

Jill and me 1967,

1984 benefit,

Boys,

chip's family,

Groeger family,

2005 Christmas card

dad and mom,

uncle Bill Iwo Jima,

football,

all County basketball,

Margie and uncle Phil,

1984 benefit p. 2,

boys #2,

Tucker,

6 lb. Cutthroat,

last picture of 4 boys.

Dad young Marine,

freshman dance 1963,

all County football,

basketball 1966,

Kathleen

Houston Astros chip

me in Barbados,

Ty

Colorado reflections

CHAPTER 13
Trials and Tribulations of Multiple Sclerosis and Other Important Stuff

The multiple sclerosis had stolen my life away in chunks, some small ones, and some big ones. Anything that caused me stress, like a cold, kidney stones, a heart attack, a dentist appointment, a UTI, a failing business, or government intervention, took another chunk out of me. My legs were gone, my left hand was useless, and my right hand only functioned a little. Fortunately, I could still breathe, talk, and think. If not for my Kathleen, I would be in a nursing home. I used to do 10,000 things, and now I could do a hundred. It was the things I could do that I focused on, not the things I couldn't.

I really have tried to tell you my history. Hopefully, it's been educational and entertaining. There is more that I'd like to share, mostly about living with multiple sclerosis, but also my own thoughts and ideas about multiple sclerosis and life. I know I have been blessed with my Kathleen and my four boys.

This chapter will be a combination of information about treatments and medications, and my feelings about multiple sclerosis and just a lot of things in general.

From the time I was diagnosed, I always felt that I would not get worse. I expected I'd either stay the same, or get better. I had heard stories of multiple sclerosis sufferers who suddenly got better, and I just knew that would happen to me.

I didn't think of myself as a bad person before my diagnosis, but I became a better person afterward. I had always believed in God. I felt he had helped me many times before and would help me again.

Being in Colorado Springs, the Christian capital of the country, it should have been easy finding God. Our closest neighbors were Christians and worked with Athletes in Action. He would come over and talk to me about Jesus. We even started a Bible reading night with another neighbor, and I was really getting into it.

This fellow, Gary, told me that he read Proverbs every morning. Whatever the date was, he would read the chapter in Proverbs whose number corresponded to that day of the month. I started doing that, too. On the ninth day of the month, I would read Proverbs 9. I was watching a lot of Christian television and went to several churches to have hands laid upon me.

The first invitation I received to attend a church came from a customer of the Chevrolet dealership, who told me he was sure I would be healed. Kathleen and I went to the service, and it was the first time that either one of us had heard people speaking in tongues. The person who invited us should have explained about the service and the church, because we were really freaked out when we left. The customer invited us back the next night, assuring me that this would be the night I would be healed.

When the minister made the call to people to come to the front to accept Jesus as their Lord and savior, I went to accept the Lord, and Kathleen followed me. The faith healer's name was Harry Hills. I was the only person in a wheelchair at the service, and Mr. Hills invited me to the front and asked if I wanted God to heal me. I said yes.

People started praying in tongues and laying hands on me. Right in the middle of all this, the customer from the dealership came up and said that Jesus had talked to him and said that tomorrow night would be the night I'd be healed.

We had plans to go fishing that night up in the mountains, and Kathleen said that we would be closer to God in the mountains than in that church. The services were held in a building that had been a roller rink prior to becoming a church. They were truly the holy rollers. I had to agree with Kathleen, and we went fishing.

One of Kathleen's coworkers invited us to her church one night, because they were having a faith healer. This was a big, well-known church in town. We met Susie at the church. I've forgotten the name of the minister, but he was laying hands on a lot of people. When he asked who else wanted to be healed, I raised my hand, but he just went past me to someone else.

Soon the service ended, and Susie was quite upset that the minister hadn't seen me. She searched the building for him so he could see me. When she finally found him and asked if he would see me, he said he would. Susie took me to him. He started praying and asking God to help me. He prayed over me for some time. When he finished, he asked me how I felt. I didn't feel any difference, but he asked me to keep in touch with him.

Several other times people just stopped me on the street to pray for me. I really didn't mind this at all. I had always been taught that praying was a good thing.

As time goes by and you don't get any better, you kind of accept the fact that you're not going to improve, so you better start living your life the best you can. Many people have told me they could never do what I do. I don't believe that. They just haven't found themselves in my situation.

It would be easy to give up, but you always need to have hope and faith. Whenever mine starts to fade, I always hear Jill's voice in my head, saying, "I knew that he would take the easy way out."

I had an Indian friend who explained their belief about suicide. The Indians ask, "Why would you want to go to a place where you're not invited?"

It's written in the Bible that suicide is a sin and sends you to hell. I once heard someone say that maybe there is no hell, but why would you take a chance?

There are plenty of reasons to keep going. I don't think that giving up is in my nature, no matter what Jill says.

◆   ◆   ◆

That would be a good segue into my next story. In the fall of 2000, I got a call from Kane, my oldest son. He told me that in November, 2001, he was getting married. I had thought for sure he was going to be a bachelor all his life, since he was already past thirty. Kane is six feet one inch tall, like me, and if it wasn't for his prematurely gray hair, we could almost be twins.

Kathleen and I started making plans to be in Boston for the wedding. Then Kane informed me that there would not be any children allowed at the wedding. Of course, I went off the deep end. We rarely go anywhere without Ty and Tucker, and we naturally wanted to take them to their brother's wedding. Mark wasn't invited either, which didn't seem right. I just could not understand Kane.

Kathleen took hold of me and said, "Let's not make waves. This is Kane's wedding, and you certainly don't want to cause trouble in your relationship with him now."

Once again, Kathleen was right, so we started making plans for the two of us to drive to Boston. As the wedding date got closer, we asked Kathleen's sister, Lynne, if she wanted to make the trip with us. She agreed to go to Boston with us. You might wonder how I could travel two thousand miles with two women, especially sisters, but I had traveled with Kathleen and Lynne several times before. We've have had our moments, but we always got along.

I wasn't too concerned about the trip, except that it was only two months after 9/11. My big concern was Kane's mother, Jill. I had not actually talked to her in twenty-five years. Kathleen was a little hesitant about meeting my ex-wife, and so was Lynne.

When we got to Boston, Kane invited us to his house for a take-out dinner. Everyone got along, and Jill was a peach. We told stories from the past, and we laughed. I met my new daughter-in-law, Kate, who was just a doll.

The wedding was held in an old mansion in the Back Bay section of Boston. During the reception, I saw a lot of Jill's relatives I hadn't seen in a long time, including her mother, sister, and brother. I had a good time, and I think Kathleen did, too. The appetizers were very Boston: clams, oysters on the half shell, and crab puffs. And of course, the cocktails flowed. The meal was an excellent filet mignon. I met a lot of Kane's friends from work and college, and also met Kate's family.

Since Lynne was not attending the wedding, she had planned to meet a friend in Connecticut. Kathleen and I had plans to go to New Jersey after the wedding. Kane and Kate were going to Jamaica for their honeymoon.

Kathleen and I drove to Mystic Seaport to pick up Lynne. She was visiting an old friend of the family. Kathleen and I called him Honus, which really wasn't his name, but it kept us amused for the rest of the trip. Honus brought Lynne to Mystic Seaport, and we had lunch with him there before we headed to New Jersey.

All in all, it was a great trip. I even got a chance to talk with Jill. We talked over a lot of things that had happened way back when.

We also had a great time in New Jersey. Kathleen met a lot of my friends, and we spent time with Aunt Margie and Uncle Phil. After two weeks, we had to head back to Colorado.

◆   ◆   ◆

I think stem cell research is exciting and may result in help for a lot of people. But I'm sure it's a few years in the future, especially because of the controversy over embryos. Still, a lot of things have happened in the past forty years or so concerning the disabled. The Vietnam veterans who came back disabled also came back mad. They had gone off to a war they didn't want to fight. It was a war with no just cause, except maybe a political one. There had been no Pearl Harbor or World

Trade Center bombing to get the country's patriotic juices flowing. These guys were sent to a country to fight without being given a clear-cut reason. I was in high school during the early years of Vietnam, and I remember a friend of mine graduating, going off to Vietnam, and not coming home. His family lived across the street, and his mother put a symbol in the window representing his passing. I always wanted to go and talk to his mother and father, but I never did. He was the first person I knew from my county to die in the war.

The disabled Vietnam veterans came home feeling the country really owed them something. They were instrumental in getting changes made. Without them, the Americans with Disabilities Act probably would not exist. The ADA was written with the best of intentions, and it had great possibilities for the future of disabled people. Unfortunately, the Americans with the disabilities are the only ones who take it seriously.

◆   ◆   ◆

As long as there are diseases, wars, car accidents, sports injuries, and alcohol and drug abuse, there will be a need for wheelchairs. It infuriates me when people who are not disabled use the disabled parking spots. I need five feet to lower the lift on my van and get in or out. When I worked at the mall, I tried to park in a van-accessible spot with at least five feet alongside it, marked off in yellow stripes, for exactly that purpose. Someone else always felt they needed that spot more than I did. Occasionally, the car had a disabled plate or placard, but more times than not, someone just wanted a closer place to park. At one time, the city hired disabled folks to police such things. Apparently that didn't work, because they now use a police car marked Disability Parking Patrol.

I'd like to see questions about disability parking on the drivers' license test, but it'll probably never happen. I always thought that Colorado Springs was a progressive town, but my hometown in New Jersey, which is probably a hundred years older, seems to have complied better with the ADA. It seems that curb cuts and ramps are a major problem for the city planners. Things are improving, but they still need a lot of training. One day I pulled into a handicap parking spot, got out, and looked for the ramp. I had to laugh, because it was right in the middle of the parking place. Of course, with the van parked in the space, I couldn't get to the ramp. I would have had to get back into the van and back up four feet to reach the ramp.

One time, Kathleen and I had a problem with sales tax on a handicapped-equipped vehicle we had purchased. We had to go to city hall, to a city council meeting. There was a handicapped parking spot just outside the front door, and we parked in it. But the spot had a parking meter that only allowed twenty minutes. In the middle of the meeting, Kathleen had to excuse herself to feed the meter. All the other meters were good for up to two hours.

We pointed this out to the city employees during our meeting. The next time we went to City Hall, the handicapped parking place was gone. They remedied the situation, just not in the way we expected. It kills me that people who are not disabled or in a wheelchair don't understand. I would never wish for anyone else to need a wheelchair, but these people just don't have a clue. For a while, they put executives in wheelchairs for a day, so they would know how it felt. It sounded like a good idea. Unfortunately, when you know you can get up and walk away from your wheelchair, there's quite a difference. I have been sitting on my butt for more than twenty years now, and it is not fun. But you do what you have to do to get through life.

The disabled have also had a lot of influence on wheelchair technology, especially powered chairs. In the last twenty years, they have come a long way. The chair I use now does nearly anything I want or need. With the help of a new environmental control unit, I can dial and answer the phone, open doors, and control the television. It does pretty much anything a remote control can do.

The whole thing comes down to the squeaky wheel getting the grease. It used to be that anyone with a disability was shoved into the background and ignored. Remember when everything possible was done to keep from showing President Franklin Roosevelt in a wheel-chair? Maybe he could have done more for the disabled, but he was in the middle of a war and depression.

Okay, I'll get off my soapbox now. But at least you know my feelings on the subject. I agree that the handicapped world has come a long way, but there's still a lot more to be accomplished.

◆   ◆   ◆

When Kathleen and I met, we both were starting fresh. She was just out of school, and I had just gone into a wheelchair. We learned things together. Shortly after we met, I asked her to take me to the gym to shoot some baskets. I was having a little trouble with my strength, so I asked her to roll me in for a lay-up. As she rolled me in for the shot, I was watching the ball to see if it went in. I found myself on the floor because Kathleen had stopped the chair. She helped me back into my chair, and we laughed.

Not long after that, we were going to go swimming at the pool at the apartment, and Kathleen was pushing me down a grassy knoll. It wasn't real steep, but it was steep enough. It was a good thing it was grassy, because she stopped, and I fell out of the chair.

One day I was in my power chair at home, and I felt my body begin to spasm. No one else was home, so I pulled my chair up against the couch to try to keep myself from falling out. It didn't work, and I found myself sliding to the floor. The chair was too close to the couch, and I got stuck. As I reached back to grab the joystick, the chair moved, and I fell to the floor in a heap. The pain was tremendous, and I was sure I'd broken something.

I finally got flat on the floor and dragged myself toward the phone. I pulled on the wire, and the phone fell to the floor. I dialed Kathleen's sister, Lorie, who was living just down the street. I explained my predicament and asked her to call Kathleen. She did, and then came up to the house. She checked both my legs, and neither one was broken. Soon Kathleen showed up, and they tried to pick me up, but could not. At the time, we didn't have a Hoyer lift, but Kathleen had seen a policeman down at the end of the block. She went to see if he would help, and the three of them got me back in the chair.

I've told you these three stories to make a point: Always wear your seat belt!

◆   ◆   ◆

The medical profession really doesn't know much about multiple sclerosis, except that it affects everyone differently. They think it's a virus that stays dormant in your system until something traumatic happens in your life. That makes sense to me, since several people that I've known had some kind of problem, then soon developed symptoms. Something like my back operation seems to bring on multiple sclerosis. The father of a friend of mine with MS was convinced that the disease came from a vaccination. Maybe he's right. His son was a little younger than me, a schoolteacher and a good-looking, athletic guy. When his MS got really bad, they had to move him into a nursing home, and I'm sorry to say that he died there.

Kathleen has promised me that she will never put me in a nursing home. I thank God for that. Lately there's been quite a lot on television about what goes on in nursing homes. Most of them are not good places to be.

Slurred speech, numbness, weakness, double vision, lack of strength, or a dragging leg can all be symptoms of multiple sclerosis. In some patients, the condition stays about the same, some people get worse gradually, and sometimes someone gets better. When I was first diagnosed, there wasn't much available in the way of treatment. Now there are all types of new programs. There seems to be a new celebrity announcing they have MS every few months. Some of them include Terry Garr, an actress; Montel Williams, a talk-show host; Annette Funicello, the Mickey Mouse Club girl; Jimmy Huga, an Olympic skier; and David L. Lander, the actor who played Squiggy on the Laverne and Shirley Show. Even the great comedian, Richard Pryor, who said, "God gave me this disease to save my life," has been diagnosed with MS. He feels the disease was sent to save him from his drug and alcohol abuse.

Everyone copes with their diagnosis and symptoms in their own way. Jimmy Huga is convinced that exercise is the answer. I tend to agree with him. When I was young and very active in sports, my symptoms were few and far between. However, when I stopped being active, the symptoms came fast and furious. I tried to exercise after the symptoms started, but it just made them worse. Now I don't try to exercise anymore. When I was only having a little trouble walking, I would go to an athletic club. They had a lap pool where I could walk in the water. After a few laps, I'd be so tired and weak, I couldn't get out of the pool without help. I also tried ankle weights. I would sit on the edge of the bed and just work my lower legs. It really tired me out, and I couldn't do much for the rest of the day. I finally came to the conclusion that exercise is only good to a point. You have to know what your limits are, and when to quit. I also tried a lot of weird stuff like pineapple concentrate supplements. These came from Hawaii and were awfully expensive. Ultimately, they did nothing for me. I took multivitamins and drank shakes for over a year, at a cost of $150 to $200 per month. At least they did something. I lost twenty pounds. I also developed a lovely kidney stone from the calcium.

I've always said that if putting a banana in my ear would help, I would do it. Each case study uses a placebo. As a participant, you either take the real medicine or a sugar tablet. People are amazed when they hear that someone who got the placebo improved. I say if it helps, who cares what it is?

CHAPTER 14
Multiple Sclerosis—The Lighter Side

HOT AND COLD

This disease has its own way of operating, and an MS patient can't let his or her body's core temperature get too high or too low. At either extreme, movement becomes difficult. I've learned to find shade as soon as possible in the summer. The heat just drains my energy. I can feel it fading away as my body gets warmer. A hat with a brim, like a baseball cap, really helps. I avoid the direct sun.

Humidity is a problem, too. With high humidity, it doesn't matter whether or not you're in the sun. The good thing about living in Colorado is that the humidity is almost always low. The last time we visited New Jersey during the summer, we went to the Jersey Shore. The humidity had to be nearly one hundred, and the temperature was close to that, too. I think I might have died if it hadn't been for the many air-conditioned bars along the boardwalk. There's nothing better than an icy cold beer to cool down that core temperature.

The cold doesn't sap my energy like the heat does; it just makes it really difficult for me to move. There have been times when I couldn't operate my chair because I got too cold. It also seems to affect my bladder control.

Kathleen has found that putting a coat or jacket on me backward is not only easy for her, but easier on me. The chair keeps my back warm, so I'm just as warm that way. It looks a little like I'm in a straight jacket, but I've gotten used to the stares.

I remember way back when I saw Dr. Parks, he said to take cool showers and let him know if that helped with the numbness. I didn't try it then because it seemed to me that using cold water defeated the purpose of taking a shower. Of course, since then I've found out that a cool or lukewarm shower really does help. When I was still walking, I got into a Jacuzzi, then couldn't understand why I felt so tired and drained. I certainly stay away from hot water now.

Being nervous or excited makes things difficult, too. When I'm trying to get out of the van by using the lift, and people are watching, I have more difficulty negotiating the chair. I become tongue tied easily and find it difficult to express myself.

◆   ◆   ◆

At one point, when Kathleen's sister, Beth, was attending the University of Colorado at Colorado Springs, she asked me if I would talk to her class about being disabled. I agreed and outlined a short presentation. When I practiced my talk on Kathleen, it was only about ten minutes long. Then Beth asked if I could talk for forty-five minutes to an hour. I took my outline along, thinking I would wing it. Before I knew it, the professor was telling me that if I wanted a question and answer period, I would have to stop. I had rambled for over an hour.

This took place pretty early in the progression of my disease, and I was still driving with the use of hand controls. I was in a manual chair. The talk went well, and the students seemed to enjoy it. I can remember trying impress on them that a disabled person lived within boundaries that they, themselves, never even noticed. I told a few funny stories that got their attention, and illustrated my point. The question and answer period was also pretty interesting. The students had some good questions and, of course, some wiseass questions, but they were young college students, and I took it with a grain of salt.

SEX

From the time of my diagnosis, I had read and been told that things were going to get tough sexually. I don't know why, but for me it happened later rather than sooner. When Kathleen and I were married, things were still working pretty well, and we had two sons.

However, the past few years have been a different story. Low libido and erectile dysfunction are big obstacles to overcome. Fortunately, new products and drugs seem to come out at the most opportune time. Viagra is a great example. When I first took Viagra, I felt like I was sixteen again. Now they're coming out with even more potent types of drugs. Again, it is just in time, because the Viagra has lost all of the benefit it gave me in the past. Levitra and Cialis are the two new drugs that sound promising.

My desire to be with Kathleen sexually has diminished quite a bit. I love her more than ever, but the problem is low libido. This has been my biggest disappointment about the progression of my MS.

I recently heard that they are working on a new drug in the form of a nose spray. Unlike Viagra or the other drugs that directly affect the penis, this medication works within the brain and affects the portion that controls the sex drive. The drug is only in the testing phase, so it will probably be a couple of years before it hits the market.

When you can't move too well, sex can be difficult. It takes creativity, but, along with the help of penile dysfunction drugs, it's possible to get things done for your partner, not to mention yourself.

At one point, with a friend's help, I purchased a device I thought might help our situation. I wasn't sure how Kathleen would feel about using it. She said it was sweet of me to be so concerned about her, but that was about as far as it ever went.

KIDS

It took my kids a long time to understand I was not like other fathers. Tucker is twelve and Ty is fifteen, so by this time they can understand why I'm different. That's not to say that they understand what my disease is all about, but I hope that they have learned something about life. Our time together has always been special. The other two boys are much older, so I'm sure that what they feel is very different.

Kane and Mark both knew me when I was still walking and not very sick. I hope they remember going fishing, playing ball, and other normal father and son activities. I know I wasn't around much when they were growing up, but I felt the time we did spend together was just for us. I'm not saying that it was all quality time, but it was healthy time.

I know Kane remembers going to softball games and doing a lot of fishing. He often talks to me about things that happened when he was a kid. I was not an ideal father, but I certainly tried my very best.

The younger boys didn't know me as a walking father. Sometimes I tell them they're lucky that I'm not walking, because I don't like little smart mouths or disrespect, especially toward their mother. Still, it is difficult to teach them to throw a ball without showing them, and it's very frustrating, too. I think the reason I keep old newspaper clippings is to show them that I could do it at one time, and it gives me some credibility when I'm trying to tell them how to do something.

Fortunately, Kathleen is very athletic, and she can go out and play catch with the boys. When Kathleen was younger, I loved to watch her play soccer and softball. She played on a few mixed leagues, and it was great when she got up to bat. The other team would yell, "Girl up," and the left fielder would move in, then would have to chase after the ball when Kathleen powered it over his head. She sure could hit that softball a long way.

I remember that at one game up in Woodland Park, she hit the ball over the fence. It was fun watching her play, and, of course, I would coach her, especially when she was in the outfield. I'd always had a sixth sense about where the batter was going to hit the ball. One time, when I was still living in New Jersey, I was asked to play with a team that was going to Delaware to play in a tournament. A big left-handed fellow was at bat, and I was playing right of center field. I just knew that this guy was going to hit the ball a long way. As soon as the ball was pitched, I started running to right field, and I mean at a dead run. I was still running when this big son-of-a gun swung the bat. He certainly got all of it, but by the time the ball got to where it was going, I was right there to catch it. The right fielder was still about thirty yards in front of me. After the game, that big batter came up to me and asked how I had caught the ball. He said he thought he'd knocked it into the next county. I told him I just knew he was going to hit it a long way.

So I would tell Kathleen where to play each batter, and, more often than not, she was in the right place to catch the ball. Unfortunately, I couldn't catch it for her. <u>I'm only kidding, Kathleen.</u> She did a great job.

◆   ◆   ◆

The younger boys really enjoy having two older brothers. They like to spend time with them when we go to New Jersey, and are always asking when we'll be going to visit or when their brothers are coming to Colorado.

I don't think that I ever used the phrase <u>half-brother</u> to the younger boys. All they know is that they have brothers. I feel that they are all part of me, and they should feel connected to each other. I hope that Mark and Kane will keep in touch with each other. When Mark was younger, he got into some trouble, and when Kane found out, he offered to help. I believe he was either still in college or had just recently graduated. I was pleased to hear that he was concerned about his brother, but I also felt he might be biting off a little more than he could chew. It wasn't a simple situation, and getting Mark out of town wouldn't have been the right solution. I just hope that as time goes by, they will grow closer.

The last time we were in New Jersey, Mark and his girlfriend invited Kane and his wife, Kate, to meet them at a local tavern for a drink. I finally thought that they might get to spend some time together, but by the time Kane and Kate got to the tavern, Mark had already left. But when Kane walked into the bar, the owner asked if he was related to me. The owner was Bonnie Petrock, and I had gone to high school with her. She was also married to my friend Howard for a while.

When they were younger, Kane and Mark used to fly to Colorado together. When Mark traveled alone, I paid extra to have an airline employee keep an eye on him, but since Kane was older, I expected him to watch out for Mark if they were on the same flight. One time Jill called, complaining that I had put too much responsibility on Kane, who was twelve or thirteen years old at the time. I tried to impress on her that they were brothers and needed to spend time together, but I don't think they ever flew together again.

Kane has a younger brother named Kyle, who Jill and Jeff had together. Kane and Kyle are close, but I really didn't get to know Kyle until Kane's wedding. I told Jill and Jeff they had done a great job raising Kyle. He is a fine young man, just like his older brother.

Mark and his three other half brothers are pretty close, too. I guess it really depends upon how kids are raised. Again, I just hope that when they are all older, and I am no longer in this world, they can rely on each other and keep in touch with each other.

DRUGS

I was never one who took many drugs, either illegal or prescription. If I had a headache and was offered an aspirin, I would say, "I don't think my body is lacking aspirin." During the '60s and '70s, drugs were always available, but since I was an athlete, I didn't use them. Beer, on the other hand, was a different story.

The drinking age in New Jersey was twenty-one. In New York, the drinking age was eighteen. We were only forty minutes from New York City and twenty from Staten Island, so we would go to Staten Island to buy our beer.

A few of my friends went off to college and changed their way of thinking. They came home doing drugs, mostly marijuana. After I graduated from high school and was out on my own, I experimented with smoking marijuana. I didn't like the way it made me feel, and shortly after smoking a joint, I would fall asleep. I could count the number of times I smoked it on one hand. Alcohol has always been my drug of choice.

Once, during my cowboy years, I met a cowgirl at a club one night, and she invited me to a cocaine party. Yes, I did try it. It was not very impressive, and I never did it again, but I vaguely remember something to do with an erection that I liked. Nose candy was not my thing.

Of course, my addiction to nicotine had a tight hold on me for many years. I never considered quitting until I met Kathleen. Tobacco was a hard addiction to kick, and I backslid a few times and started smoking again. Owning the sports bar didn't help, because everyone smoked there.

With Kathleen's help, and nicotine gum, I managed to quit. The fact that I couldn't hold or light my own cigarettes might have helped, too.

◆   ◆   ◆

Because of the disease, prescription drugs are a part of my life now. I have been through many trials and errors, trying to find the right combination to address all of my problems. During my battle with the second kidney stone, I was hospitalized. They gave me morphine for the pain, but I got a case of extreme nausea. I actually lost two days of my life, and I don't remember anything about them. Now, whenever I'm in a hospital, we always say that I am allergic to morphine, and they give me Demerol. It's pretty good and puts me directly to sleep, which serves the same purpose.

Good old Dr. Bell, when he first put me in the hospital, treated me with ACTH, a steroid. It was administered intravenously, and I don't remember if it helped. The next thing he tried was Prednisone, which was taken orally. It made me feel great and I thought that I was cured, but that feeling only lasted a couple days. All the other times I took it, it only made me retain water and then urinate more. Another steroid that they gave me intravenously was Solu Medrol. It didn't have any long-lasting effects for me, either.

Novantrone is a chemotherapy drug that is normally used for testicular cancer. It has recently been approved for secondary progressive MS and is supposed to retard the disease process. I was a candidate for Novantrone treatment and have had the maximum number of treatments allowed in a lifetime. It's a very toxic drug, and patients have to rinse their mouths with a solution of water and baking soda to prevent sores. Kathleen had to wear rubber gloves when handling my bowel movements and urine during the first week after the treatment.

I did notice some improvement in right hand strength and movement after the first day of the Novantrone treatment. The next day it went back to the way it had been. My neurologist feels that the treatment did its job, because a recent MRI indicated I had no new lesions in my brain. The treatments themselves really knocked me in the dirt for a week or two. I was extremely fatigued and didn't want to do anything, but because of the drug's affect on my immune system, I wasn't supposed to be around a lot of people anyway.

My primary physician, Dr. Timothy Hoke, was one of the finest doctors I have ever had the pleasure to know. Kathleen also thought there was no one better, and we were not the only patients who felt that way. Unfortunately, Dr. Hoke died in a tragic accident. Not only will his family miss him, as well as all his patients, but Colorado Springs has lost a great person.

MS can also have an effect on a patient's mental attitude, and, of course, I had this problem as well. I just did not care about anything, and I was being verbally abusive. Given my poor attitude, Dr. Hoke prescribed a new drug, Effexor. It really helps me cope, and if I don't have it, everyone knows it. I take baby aspirin and Colace, a stool softener, not to be confused with Peri-colace, which is a laxative. We did get them confused once, and it wasn't pretty. I also take an anti-spastic drug, Dantrium, which helps with leg spasms.

Here is an interesting treatment note. Someone realized that injecting Botox into tight and spastic muscles would make them loosen up and feel better. Botox is made from the germs of botulisms. I had two treatments that doctors seemed to think helped. I thought it was a good thing that I have little feeling in my arms and legs, because they stick a pretty big needle deep into your muscle. Maybe I should have had it injected into my face instead, because I'm starting to look more and more like my father. The other day, after I saw myself in the mirror naked, I told Kathleen that I looked like Mr. Burns on The Simpsons. It's an ugly thing.

Provigil is a drug normally prescribed to help patients with narcolepsy, but I take it to increase my level of alertness, since my fatigue is a big issue. It's still questionable whether it helps or not. I also take cranberry pills, which help to prevent urinary tract infections.

We always try to eliminate the drugs that don't seem to be helping in any way. The neurologist is good about not prescribing too many drugs. There are some medications that help, but they have side effects. Then there are drugs that help treat the side effects. This can go on and on and on, until the patient is taking dozens of different dr

CHAPTER 15
Adventures in Bodily Functions

NUMBER ONE: URINATION

I really didn't have a problem with urination early in the disease. Once I was diagnosed and started reading about the disease, certain things began to make more sense. At first I only experienced urgency, normally just at work. And it only became urgent once I got into the bathroom, which still gave me plenty of time to take care of things. At one time, I was prescribed Ditropan for urgency, and it was supposed to control a spastic bladder. But when I took it, I couldn't urinate at all. I went the whole day without going to the bathroom. I stopped the drug after one day.

Once I started using a manual wheelchair, my problems really increased. A lot of bathrooms have grab bars. I could still stand using the grab bars. The problem is that while you are holding onto the grab bars, you can't hold anything else. Unless you have been blessed with an extra long member, you have difficulties with pants and underwear that always seem to be in the way. This causes you to urinate on your pants. The fact that you are sitting in a wheelchair can make that less noticeable, but you are still damp, and can be a little smelly after a time.

It didn't happen every time, but enough times to worry about it, so I used to sit in the sun for a short time after using the restroom, to allow my pants to dry a bit. One time I was attending an Easter dinner with Kathleen's family at the very fancy Broadmoor Hotel in the Springs. I was in the bathroom, trying to relieve my bladder. There were not any grab bars, but I carried a plastic urinal just in case. While

I was in there, an older, well-dressed gentleman came in. He noticed my plight and he spent twenty minutes telling me about his prostate problems.

As time went on and transferring to the toilet or standing became more difficult, the use of the plastic urinal became the norm. Again, as things progressed, using the urinal became more and more difficult, especially with the urgency factor and the decreased hand function. Getting to your zipper and grabbing the member you need to urinate with requires fine motor skills that I no longer had. I needed a new solution to the urination problem. Of course, Kathleen, being in the medical field, found the answer. We soon became familiar with a Texas, or condom, catheter, but there was a trial-and-error period. This device is very similar to a condom or prophylactic, except that there's a hose at one end and the urine should flow into a bag attached to your leg. The device attaches to your penis like a condom with glue on it, and you have to find the size that fits you best. You also have to be aware of how much you may have voided, because if you overflow the bag, the urine backs up and the glue comes loose. Then you have wet pants, a wet wheelchair seat, and a wet floor. Overflowing became a real problem once I could not empty the bag by myself.

When I had the gift shop, the help would empty the bag for me. I had to buy rubber gloves for the girls, which was only fair. Dee Dee didn't enjoy this job, and she got very angry if she was emptying the bag and I had to go some more. She just didn't understand that I had no control over the matter. When I owned the sports bar, a few of my friends would help me, and some of the employees would help, too.

Lack of fluids causes urinary tract infections [UTI]. After I sold the sports bar and was at home by myself, I would limit my intake of fluids to prevent overflow. But it would still happen, and Kathleen would have to come home, clean me up, and change my pants and underwear. That got old real fast, so I limited my fluid intake even more, and my UTI became more common. The infections would really make me sick, which made the MS worse. We needed another quick solution.

Good old Kathleen came to the rescue once again. After much research, she found a device that would empty the bag when I pressed a button attached to my chair. With this new device, I could drink as much water as I needed. But, again, nothing is absolutely foolproof. There were times when I forgot to empty the bag, causing overflow. A couple of times, the bag wasn't hooked up right and wouldn't drain, causing overflow. Occasionally Kathleen forgot to take the little cap off the emptying device. Yep, causing overflow.

Now that we've had this device for a few years, accidents are few and far between. I drink a certain amount of water every day, and I know when to empty the bag. I can empty the bag outside in the grass, or, during bad weather, I can empty it in the roll-in shower.

I can hear you thinking, <u>And what about nighttime? What do you do then?</u> Funny you should ask. Nighttime could be a problem because the leg bag only holds 1000 cc, and there could be a lot of overflow. The solution for that problem is a night drain bag. It has longer tubing, and lies on the floor.

At one point, I had such frequent urinary tract infections that the urologist was considering a supra-pubic catheter. This is a tube inserted surgically, directly into the bladder just above the pubic bone. Fortunately, he decided to keep trying the condom catheter. I started taking cranberry additives, which seemed to help fight off infections in the urinary tract. The continued use of the condom catheter suited me fine. In my opinion, once they start putting tubes into your body, things aren't going well.

I spoke briefly about my friend, Bob, who was a teacher with MS. When they put him in a nursing home, he had problems with his bowel program. They operated on him, did a colostomy, and not long after that, he passed away. I'm sure that certain procedures are helpful, but I still wouldn't want them done to me.

NUMBER TWO: BOWEL MOVEMENT
<u>or</u> "MA, PA CRAPPED HIMSELF!"

The number two bodily function is something which everyone calls Number Two, but if you have an accident with Number Two, it quickly becomes your number one priority. It certainly is a lot messier than a Number One accident, and smells worse, too. And you can't cure it by sitting in the sun for a while before you go back to work.

One time while I was working at the Chevrolet dealership, I found myself in a bad situation. The dealership had installed grab bars at the urinal in the bathroom off the showroom, but there was no wheelchair-accessible toilet. The mechanics' bathroom was large, with four stalls, but none of them were wheelchair-accessible, either. I was still standing up back then, and I would park my wheelchair at the open stall door and stand. Then I'd grab onto the stall partition and work my way backward to the toilet. Once I reached the toilet, I would hold onto the stall partition with one hand, and pull my pants down with the other hand. Then, naked from the butt down, I would make a very delicate pivot to sit on the toilet. When I was done, I would use toilet paper. After I flushed the toilet, I would dip some more toilet paper in the water and use it to wipe my butt between my legs. I know this does not sound very hygienic, but you have to do what you have to do.

This particular day, I was all done and started to stand, reaching up for the stall partition to hold onto while I pulled up my underwear and pants. All of a sudden, I realized I was not finished, and I tried to pivot back to the toilet. I missed the toilet's center, and as I was lowering myself, I had another bowel movement, which landed right where I was lowering myself to sit. Needless to say, I had a huge mess all over myself, and I couldn't get it cleaned off. After I got my underwear and pants up, I was really a mess. It would have been a tough thing for me to try to explain to my bosses, but fortunately, Chip was there and handled things. I took the rest of the day off. I was still living at my mother's, and she had the misfortune of helping me clean myself up.

At least I was still mobile enough to get in and out of the shower by myself.

Fortunately, that type of accident rarely happened at work. I asked Mr. Williams if he could make one of the stalls in the mechanics' bathroom wheelchair-accessible. I believe he looked into it, but cost became a factor, and it was never done.

As time went on and I got physically worse, the problems of bowel movements just increased. During my time at the souvenir store, nearly every time I bent over in my chair to pick something up, I would have an accident. Dee Dee started calling me Mister Mister Poopy Pants. She was so kind. I couldn't sit around in my own feces for long before I started to smell, so I'd go home and wait for Kathleen to come home and help me. As you can see, Number Two can be more important than Number One.

As I mentioned in the drug segment, I take Colace, which is a stool softener. When the doctor initially suggested I take it, Kathleen went to the grocery store and picked some up. Suddenly, I was having an accident every day, and we couldn't understand what the problem was. When Kathleen read the instructions on the bottle, she realized she had purchased Peri-colace, which is a laxative. We quickly corrected that problem.

One of the unfortunate things about having MS is that I don't have any clue when I'm about to have an accident. It could be caused by something I've eaten. One day, while I was sitting at home, I felt as though I had a little gas. It turned into a full-blown case of diarrhea. It was early in the afternoon, and I tried not to call Kathleen at work, since she is always so busy with patients and hospital stuff. But Ty was home.

I thought I could tough this one out and wait until Kathleen got home from work. Well, this was about the worst diarrhea I'd ever had. The smell was unbelievable, and the backs of my legs started to burn. I asked Ty if he would call his mother and see if she was really busy or might be coming home anytime soon. Kathleen, in her infinite wisdom, knew something was up. She asked Ty what was wrong, and he said, "Ma, Pa crapped himself!"

Kathleen thought that was the funniest thing she had ever heard. She still laughs if the story is mentioned. Nevertheless, she came home to clean me up. The diarrhea was pretty toxic, and my legs were already turning red, so it was a good thing that we called her. Since then, she's made us promise not to hesitate and to call her immediately.

It seemed to take a long time to set up my bowel program, but we've been on the same one for a couple of years now, and it seems to be working quite well. Digital Stim, Dulcolax, Mod, Max, and Min are some of the pleasant terms that we have learned. And don't forget about suppositories. They are a necessity in a bowel program. Having something stuck up my butt is not my favorite experience. Then there's digital stimulation. They should call it The Finger, and it certainly isn't pleasant either. Since I've had these bowel program experiences, I know I could never have been gay. Mod, for moderate, Max, for maximal, and Min, for minimal, are all terms that describe the amount of whatever you're doing at the time.

OTHER MISCELLANEOUS BODILY FUNCTIONS

There are other things that people take for granted that cause me serious problems. A runny nose that cannot be wiped clean or blown becomes a major sniffing episode. After a while you start to feel backed up in the nose area, and you figure there might be a problem. I tell Kathleen I have a floater. It usually happens while she's brushing my teeth. I can use a power toothbrush with help from Kathleen, but if I can't breathe, then I realize that there's something stuck up there. Kathleen leans me forward toward the sink, and I blow the boogie out of my nose. When I occasionally blow an exceptional one, she puts it on a Kleenex and runs around the house showing the boys the gigantic boogie that their father has cultivated. Then she comes back to the bathroom to tell me how disgusting I am. As you see, she gets a big kick out of the whole thing.

Another issue that becomes important is cleaning my ears. I cannot hold a Q-tip in either hand, and if I did get hold of one, I would probably jam it into my brain. Unless I remind Kathleen, my ears don't get cleaned. I waited so long last summer that I lost part of the hearing in my left ear, which came in handy when I didn't want to listen to someone. It had been bothering me for a couple weeks before Kathleen asked Lynne, the physician's assistant, to check out my ear. She started flushing the ear out with warm water, using one of those suction things made for babies. After a few minutes I heard a pop, and heard Kathleen scream, "Oh, that is disgusting!" A large piece of wax had come out of my ear, and I could hear again. Kathleen always seems to be screaming or laughing a lot, which keeps the situation light. I wouldn't have it any other way, and that's one of the reasons why I love her so much.

Scratch your ear when it itches. Pull the covers up after you crawl into bed. Comb your hair, if there's any left. Dress yourself in the morning. These are all things that able-bodied folks take for granted, and they're necessary daily functions that I can't perform for myself anymore. My disease has worsened pretty drastically in the past several years, but when I think about it, I realize it took me a long time to get to this point. I know I'm repeating myself, but if it were not for Kathleen, I would be in a nursing home today. I know Chip could not do what Kathleen does for me. Nor would I want him to, even if he were willing to try. A good core support system is mandatory if you're going to live with this disease. I have been so very fortunate to have had bosses, friends, and relatives who were willing and able to support me.

Then, of course, there is my Kathleen Marie. There is no one else like her. When I tell her she must be getting sick of this, because I am sick and tired of the whole situation, she says that she'll continue to do what she does because she loves me. Now, how great is that?

ATROPHY

I never had big legs or arms, but after limited exercise for twenty years, my legs and arms have atrophied to mere skin and bone. I had a normal behind, not too big, not too small, and the girls liked it. Now there is nothing left after sitting on it for twenty years. It's an ugly site. A recent MRI showed my spinal cord has also atrophied. I guess what Kathleen says is true: if you don't use it, you lose it.

MIGRAINE HEADACHES

Back when my brother and I owned a business together, I suddenly got a dull headache one afternoon. It was nothing excruciating, just a bothersome, headachy feeling. Then I realized that I couldn't remember much of anything. Chip was getting a big kick out of asking me questions I couldn't answer. They were simple questions like my name, address, and things like that. I could think of an address or a name, but things just didn't seem to fit. This went on for an hour or two, and then, just as fast as it started, it ended. It was over so quickly, I didn't seek medical treatment or advice.

After that, the same thing happened quite a few times. Kathleen decided she'd better tell Dr. Hoke about it. He said it sounded like a migraine headache, and unless it hurt, not to worry too much about it. He did give me some Midrin to take if it happened again. And, of course, the last time it happened, I was alone. I couldn't get to the medication, so I just rode it out.

BEACH TRANSFER

One of Kathleen's favorite transfers is the beach transfer. The patient must be in a manual wheelchair. Using the push handles, Kathleen would lay the chair back to the floor, then roll the patient's legs out of the chair. This would leave the patient flat on the floor.

One day I was at the hospital waiting for Kathleen for lunch. She was treating a guy in a manual chair and working on his arms. All of a sudden he became non-responsive. Thinking quickly, Kathleen performed a beach transfer and saved the guy's life. She has done that move on me many times to get me on the floor. Kathleen, the little dickens.

BATHS OR SHOWERS

As long as I still had some function and could wash myself, showering was pretty basic. As the disease progressed and I could no longer hold soap or a washcloth, it became a little more interesting. Again, thank God for Kathleen, who handles these jobs with expertise. We try to get in one shower a week and one bed bath a week.

Cleaning certain portions of the body can get very interesting. When Kathleen is working on me, I always tell her that it is very dirty and she should spend extra time on it. She just smiles and says, "Yes darling, I know." Bed baths can also be interesting, and they are a quicker answer to a dirty problem.

CHAPTER 16
The Spices of Life:
Durable Medical Equipment

These are the things you need to get through life. As the disease progresses, these things become more and more necessary. None of them are cheap, and some of them can get quite expensive. Insurance, Medicare, and Medicaid will help with some things.

AFOs

AFO stands for ankle foot orthosis. When I was still walking, I dragged my left foot. After I started using crutches, I had trouble swinging my left foot through for the next step. As my physical therapist, Kathleen suggested that a pair of AFOs might help me. That first pair was off the shelf and weren't fitted to me, but they worked just fine for a while. After I was in a wheelchair, the AFOs prevented dropped foot. About this time, I had form-fitting braces made, and I still wear them every day.

CRUTCHES

There are all types of crutches, including the old wooden ones and the new aluminum style. There are loft strand or Canadian crutches, which was what I used. Kathleen's sister, Lynne, is comfortable using the old wooden crutches. She had polio as a child and gets along very well on them.

SHOWER CHAIRS AND COMMODES

Some wheelchairs can go into the shower. For the more mobile, they make stationary chairs that sit in the shower. There are also chairs that can be used as toilets, or commodes. An extra tall toilet can make transfers easier.

HOYER LIFT

This little wonder has been a Godsend around our house. Most of the time, Kathleen could physically transfer me from my chair to the bed and from the bed to my chair. But ever since my heart attack, transferring has been nearly impossible without help.

There have been times when Kathleen's back hurt, and she would use the Hoyer lift. I use the same chair for both showering and Number Two. Because it is lower, Kathleen has trouble physically transferring me, and she uses the Hoyer lift for that, too.

One time, I decided to get on the floor for some reason, and we had one hell of a time trying to get me back into my chair. After a lot of laughing and grunting, Kathleen used the Hoyer lift.

WHEELCHAIRS

We have made great progress in recent years with wheelchairs. There is a wheelchair for every situation and every patient. Manual chairs are more lightweight and manageable. I remember my first manual chair and the trouble I had negotiating corners, hills, and doorways. My knuckles were bloody most of the time.

Getting up hills does take a lot of strength, but it also takes practice, just like anything else. When my boys would come to me and say they couldn't do something, I would say, "You just have to practice, and you'll be able to do it." If you're confined to a wheelchair and hills are a problem, there are Hill Holders that will prevent the chair from rolling backward as you're going up the hill.

Tucker came home one day and said he was having trouble in gym. He was having a heck of a time jumping rope the way the teacher wanted him to. We went outside with the jump rope, and he started to jump. After explaining what the teacher wanted, I told him to practice. It didn't take him long to become the best jump-roper in his class. After many years in a manual wheelchair, anyone becomes proficient. It just takes practice!

There are now wheelchairs for people who can only use one hand, like a stroke patient. Sports chairs and racing chairs are popular with the athletic folks. Olympics for the disabled and wheelchair patients are very popular. Some people really get into their fancy wheelchairs.

Penrose Hospital recently hired a new physiatrist, a doctor of rehabilitation. Dr. Glen House is in a wheelchair, and I believe he is a quadriplegic. He's a great doctor, especially for wheelchair patients. He is my doctor now, and I know from personal experience that it is very satisfying to talk to a doctor who knows what you're going through.

Recently, Dr. House was involved in a promotional campaign to prevent head injuries. He climbed Pike's Peak using the highway, but in a new type of chair. This chair can calculate the amount of pressure needed to move up an incline. Once the chair makes that calculation, it will move up the incline when the occupant exerts the same amount of strength needed to move the chair on a flat surface.

Dr. House made the twelve-mile trek to the top of America's mountain in record wheelchair time, mostly on a dirt road. A group of climbers went up the mountain on Barr Trail and found that the good doctor had beaten everybody to the summit.

POWER WHEELCHAIRS

There have been twice as many advances in power chairs in the past few years. The old power chairs were slow and unreliable and considered a luxury. When Kathleen noticed I was having difficulty getting up the driveway and ramp to the house, she suggested I get a power chair. Before, she had always said, "If you don't use it, you will lose it."

But because of the difficulties I was encountering, she decided it was time for a power chair. I had seen a chair at our local rehab equipment store that looked like a little tank with four small, thick wheels. It just looked like it would be good outdoors. We were still doing a lot of fishing, and this chair looked like it wouldn't have any trouble getting me where I wanted to go. It was an Arrow XT, manufactured by Invacare, which is a pretty reputable company that's been around a long time. The chair did what I thought it would do.

Power chairs are normally operated with the use of a joystick, similar to the ones on video games. I was having difficulty making right-hand turns with my joystick. Even after they adjusted the sensitivity, I still couldn't do it. The problem was always worse later in the day, when I got tired. They suggested that I would do better with a head control, which was true. We also considered a chin control, but that was really for someone who had little head movement. There is even a control called a sip and puff, which has a tube that goes into your mouth. The patient controls the chair by blowing and sucking on the tube. This device is great for people who cannot move at all. I believe I saw Christopher Reeves, the actor who played Superman, using that particular control.

As far as chair functions go, the new generation of controls can tilt the chair in space, recline it, and move the footrests up and down. The seat can be raised or lowered to help with reaching things. These functions are usually operated with buttons or toggle switches. They now have a voice activated system control, too. Hopefully, I'll be able to get one, which sure would make things easier.

After my heart attack, Kathleen suggested that I get a wheelchair that would recline. We ordered another XT with a La-Bac recline system. According to insurance company and government guidelines, a power wheelchair has a lifetime of five years, so every five years you can get a new chair. The other way they'll let you get a new chair is if you develop more medical problems.

One day while I was at the sports bar, the rep from our local rehab equipment store brought a new chair in to show me. It was called a Permobil and was made in Sweden. The chair was much smaller than my XT, had front-wheel-drive, and also had a recline system. I really liked the chair, and it was about time to get a new one, so we bought it. It was a great chair, and I loved being in it. As a matter of fact, I still keep it as my backup chair.

Not long ago, I started having trouble with my butt. It stayed sore and bruised no matter what we did. The Permobil Company had added a new feature to their chairs that allowed the chair to tip from side to side, and it was just the solution to my problem. So I got a new Permobil, and my butt has never been better.

You'll really need to practice operating your power chair, even more than a manual one. These new chairs are very powerful and can knock holes in your walls and doorways. Our house is a fine example. I can't open doors with my hand, so I would just push them open with my chair or push them closed with my footrests. So, the doors look a little battered, but the doorframes and corners have been repaired. Again, practice makes perfect.

I remember one time I was going to a meeting at the mall and needed to go into a department store. My chair got caught on the doorframe, and it actually stood the chair on its back wheels. I was looking straight up at the ceiling. Fortunately, a number of helpful customers got me out of that predicament. Perhaps my nervousness about the meeting affected my ability to drive my chair that night.

Wheelchairs are much like cars, and when you get a new one, you have to get used to how it operates. It's important to train yourself to use it. Of course, the longer you've been in a chair, the shorter the training period will probably be. The new chairs can go between seven and ten miles an hour, which is pretty fast. That's much faster than a normal person walks. Of course, the faster you go, the harder it will be to control the chair.

There are always new chairs coming out. I'm sure you've heard of the chair that goes up and down stairs. I did see it, but it looks like it still needs some work. The inventor, who is not disabled, was demonstrating the chair, and he seemed to be using a lot of arm strength. This is the guy who also invented the "segway," the two wheeled machine that you stand on. It is great for people who walk a lot, like the mail man.

HANDICAPPED VANS

New vans are available almost anywhere in the States, but they aren't cheap. Even a used van can be pretty pricey. If it's too cheap, be careful, because something must be wrong with it.

I have had four handicapped vans. The first one was a 1986 Chevrolet short-bed. They don't make them anymore, because they couldn't lower the floor. Mine had a power lift, door closer, and hand controls, along with carpet and a fancy interior. I was still in a manual chair and could transfer into the driver's seat. It also had a towing package so I could pull my little boat. Working for the Chevrolet dealership, I got a great deal, but I'd only had the van for three or four years when I decided to get something newer.

The Chevrolet Astro Van was only a couple of years old. I thought it would be a good van for me. Again, I bought a conversion van before the handicapped equipment went in. Not the smart thing to do. The van had a raised roof, so putting in the power lift and door openers wasn't too much of a problem. I also had a power driver seat installed that would lift up and move back, so I could transfer. The power buttons were on the right side, so I could reach them while sitting in my chair.

I remember that several times when I was about to transfer to the driver's seat, I fell on the floor between the chair and the firewall. I couldn't get back into my chair or into the driver's seat, and I was just stuck there. Fortunately, each time I did this, Kathleen was home. I would reach up and beep the horn, and Kathleen would come out and get me up and into the driver's seat. It was a really pretty van. It was a Star Craft conversion, and they did a great job.

When I got my first power chair, I was still driving the 1988 Chevy Astro Van. It was okay for the manual chair, but the power chair is much wider, longer, and heavier. We sold the Astro Van and bought a new 1991 Ford E150, which was a conversion van. It was the wrong way to get a wheelchair-accessible van. We made every mistake, buying a van that had carpeting, captain's chairs, a fancy interior ceiling, and a lot of fancy wood trim.

I repeat: This is the wrong way to buy a wheelchair-accessible van. The right way is to buy a cargo van, and then have all the necessary work done. Lower the floor first, then have the lift installed. After that, add all the fancy stuff. Doing it the wrong way gets very expensive.

The 1991 Ford was a good vehicle, and it treated us well for over twelve years. But after a time, normal driving and trips to the east coast had pushed the odometer reading to over 120,000 miles. We decided to sell the Ford and purchase a new van.

Even though we had re-established our credit since the sports bar fiasco, I was concerned that we might have trouble securing a loan for a new vehicle. There was a place in the Springs that had a van that was perfect for my needs, but the dealer had limited financing sources. We had no luck.

I had seen an ad in one of my MS magazines for a company that only handled wheelchair-accessible vans. I checked out their website, which was very professionally done, and Kathleen and I decided that I should call them to see if we could get a new van.

I talked to one of their representatives and explained our situation. The guy was real nice and said he thought he could help us. I returned to their website to read their inventory list of new and used vans. We picked out a new van that met our needs, and the rep mailed us a brochure. The company was just like a dealership, and they handled everything. Our rep took a credit application over the phone. They had excellent financing sources, and we were approved for the loan. I was a little hesitant about the transaction, because this was the first time I had ever purchased a vehicle without seeing it.

These people were located in Minnesota, but said they would deliver our vehicle to us. The van arrived the day after my fifty-fourth birthday, and was exactly what we ordered.

I definitely recommend these people to anyone who needs a van, new or used. They will give you a fair deal. If you are interested, please go to their website, www.Rolxvans.com.

Our new van, a 2002 Ford, is dark blue. Since Kathleen does all the driving, the van has an automatic tie down where the passenger seat would be. I can roll up to the tie down and be a passenger. It's nice to ride in the front. We are ready to do more traveling.

◆   ◆   ◆

There are many places that convert wheelchair-accessible vans. There is even a company in Denver that actually manufactures them. They've done some work for us, and they are very reputable.

I have a friend, Kathy, who also has MS and is in a power chair. Her husband, Mike, is her caregiver. They were both in the Air Force.

The Veterans Administration helps Kathy quite a bit. They will pay for certain equipment in the van, along with all her health care. I met Kathy and Mike through the souvenir shop at the mall. They also used to come to the sports bar for lunch. I try to keep in touch with them, but sometimes it's a little too long before I talk to them. They live up the same mountain where Kathleen's mother lives and attend the same church as Kathleen's family. Sometimes I get information about them from Kathleen's mom.

Insurance companies and government agencies, other than the VA, feel that vans are a luxury, and they don't pay for anything.

CHAPTER 17
SHS Hall of Fame

My brother Chip cannot understand why I have such an interest in our high school days. He told me it was a long time ago and we shouldn't dwell on the past. At first I thought maybe he was right, but then I decided he wasn't. That was a time when I was normal, walking, and athletic. I believe it's good for me to see pictures of myself as I was back then. Kathleen likes those pictures, too.

When we had the sports bar, I had a few of my pictures blown up to display on the walls. She liked them so much she put them in our bedroom, on her side of the bed, after we sold the place. When I asked her if keeping the pictures around would make me seem full of myself, she said she didn't care, because she liked looking at me.

Chip got upset with me when I told him I wanted to get into the Somerville High School Hall of Fame. My oldest son told me that my friend Mark, who still lives in Somerville, was going to nominate me.

But when I started hearing who was being inducted into the Hall, I couldn't understand why they would even be considered. I asked Mark about it, and he said the whole thing was political. Rather than looking at your accomplishments during your high school years, the committee wanted to know what you'd done for the school recently. You had to have gone to college and become a teacher or an important person. If you hadn't graduated from college, you had to be All-State during high school. Mark told me that just being All-County, even in three sports, would not get me in.

The last time I was in New Jersey, I had the pleasure of visiting the high school and seeing the Hall of Fame. I recognized a lot of people who I had played sports with, but there were some names of people who either had pretty bad reputations, or who weren't even graduates of Somerville High. I really believe that someone like my father, who held a track record for over thirty-five years, and my brother, who played football and baseball and pitched a no-hitter before playing professionally, and yes, even an All-County player in three sports like me, should at least be nominated to the Hall of Fame. But that's just my opinion, and no one's listening to me.

It feels good to get that off my chest. I was pretty high up there on that soapbox, wasn't I? After all that, they would probably never let me in. But that's not a problem. Since 1967, when I graduated, they have built a new high school next to the football field, and our old high school is now a junior high. Boy, it would have been great not to have to walk that distance to practice every day. The new campus is nice. Mark's girls go there, and I think Valerie's son, Steven, went there, too.

MY KAT'LEEN

She is strong like a bull. Even now that she's getting a little older, she can still put our older boy, Ty, on the floor. He is now six feet one inch tall and weighs about 180 pounds. She still transfers me by herself, and I'm no lightweight.

Kathleen has worked at the local hospital for twenty years and is well respected there. One of her supervisors gave her the best acknowledgement. He said that he wanted it noted on his driver's license that if he was ever in an accident, Kathleen should be the physical therapist who takes care of him. She's someone who does things the right way, or she doesn't do them. Each of her patients receives one hundred percent of her attention, for however long the hospital allows her for their treatment. She goes to the hospital to work, period. She is very professional and does not slack off or push patients off onto other therapists.

My wife doesn't come home until the work is done. The hospital has been very strict lately about overtime, but because of her commitment to her patients, she still works some extra hours. But knowing hospital policy, she'll clock out, then get things done without showing overtime.

This lady is remarkable. She works a full-time job, she is a full-time caregiver to me, and she mothers two active boys…not to mention cleaning the house, doing the laundry, going grocery shopping, cooking, helping with homework, doing the lawn maintenance, watering the plants, putting up Christmas lights, taking down Christmas lights, and paying the bills. She does everything. The boys try to help somewhat now that they are older.

My wife also entertains her family often at our house. You're probably wondering what the hell I do. To be completely frank, I can't, and don't, do much. Kathleen tells me I am her support system, and she needs my help with the boys. I offer my opinion on things, whether she takes it or not.

As you can see, Kathleen has a lot on her plate, and she handles it beautifully. I know it all gets to her at times, and I try to be there for her. She's carrying a tremendous load, and sometimes I just don't know how she does it.

This is a woman who knew at an early age that she wanted to be a physical therapist. Her high school counselor told her that she would never be a therapist and should look for something else to do. When she went home and told her mother what the counselor had said, her mother told her that she could be whatever she wanted, and if she wanted to be a physical therapist, then she should become a physical therapist. And that is exactly what she did!

Being married to Kathleen is almost like having a doctor in the house. Whenever my brother has pains, he calls Kathleen. So does most everyone else in the family. My wife is well respected for her knowledge and expertise. I don't know why she stays with me, but I thank God every day that she is my Kat'leen.

BUDDY

There's another very important member of our family. His name is Buddy, and he's been with us for about nine years. He's a very active member of the family, and he is supposed to be the boys' responsibility. But Kathleen has the pleasure of taking care of him most of the time. It's just another entry on her long resume.

Buddy sleeps with Tucker and is considered Tucker's pet. He's a cute CockaPoo. He keeps me company during the daytime and is usually lying at my feet. I try to stay aware of where Buddy is so I don't run over him. On one or two occasions, I have run over him, so he's pretty alert when my chair starts to move.

About five years ago, Buddy started coughing a lot. Kathleen thought maybe he was breathing dust from the carpet, causing him to cough. We took Buddy to the vet and had an x-ray taken. Buddy had a lung tumor.

The doctor told us Buddy wouldn't live for more than a month. He could operate to remove the tumor, but the surgery would be $1,400, and he couldn't guarantee the results. We decided against the operation, basically because we didn't have an extra $1,400. Kathleen asked the doctor if she should renew Buddy's license. He said he would not renew it. We thought that we were about to lose our best friend.

Shortly after receiving the tragic news, we decided that we would pray for Buddy. One evening we put Buddy on my lap, so that all four of us could touch him. As we all laid our hands on Buddy, I prayed and asked God to help our friend.

Buddy is still with us. He coughs every once in a while, and has maybe lost a step or two. He doesn't hear as well as he used to, but he loves to chase squirrels in the back yard. When we do lose him, there will be some very sad people in our household.

CHAPTER 18
A Day in The Life...

The best way to describe my current medical status is to lead you through a normal day in my life. I know it can be difficult to visualize unfamiliar procedures and situations, so I'll try to explain everything so the inexperienced reader can understand.

6:30 A.M.

I can hear the boys getting ready for school. Ty is all ready and will head out to catch the bus. Tucker is probably looking for his breakfast or doing last-minute homework.

Kathleen has been up since 5:00 a.m. and is now doing laundry or dishes and making Tucker's breakfast. He has to leave to catch the bus at 6:45 a.m., and he's pretty loud in the mornings. About this time, Kathleen comes into the bedroom and turns the light on. We exchange our good mornings and I love yous, and she'll kiss me and prepare to get me up. She lifts the covers off me, because I can't, then goes into the bathroom to get my leg bag ready for the day. She cleans it, cleans the automatic leg bag drainer, then removes the night drain bag from my condom catheter and puts the day leg bag on. She takes the night drain bag, empties it out, and cleans it. She retrieves my wheelchair, either from being charged in the bathroom, or from the bedroom. Next she puts my pants on, careful to thread the leg bag through my pants leg. She then puts my sneakers and AFOs on, right leg first, then the left. She rolls me on my right side and moves my hips over so she can sit me up. I get to expel some gas. It's pretty sad when you don't have the muscles to fart. I have to cough or yawn to get anything out.

Kathleen physically moves my hips toward the middle of the bed. She does it so that when she sits me up, I don't slide off the bed onto the floor. She bends my legs toward my chest, and then puts my feet on the floor. My upper body is still lying on the bed, so she grabs me around the neck and sits me up. If she doesn't hold onto me, I fall backward onto the bed or forward onto the floor. As she holds me up, she reaches for the joystick on the chair to position it for the transfer. She puts her arms under my armpits, and I rest my chin on her chest. She counts to three, blocks my knees, and pivots me into the chair. I try to help by stiffening my legs. Sometimes I'm successful, but more times than not, my legs don't respond. Of course, there are days that we use the Hoyer lift, which is a lot easier on Kathleen. She doesn't like using it because it takes too long.

I am now sitting in the chair. She puts my pullover shirt on, then reclines the chair and pulls me back in the seat so I'll be comfortable. She sets the chair upright, and we head to the bathroom to brush my teeth. I can normally do it myself with an electric toothbrush, but due to a recent UTI, Kathleen has been brushing them for me. After she combs my hair, I'm off to the living room to watch the news and have my coffee. Kathleen hands me my medications and a cup of coffee, but she has to help me with the first couple of sips. Our coffee cup handles fit my two fingers, and Kathleen puts a piece of napkin between the cup and my fingers to protect me from burns.

8:00 A.M.

By 8:00, Kathleen is ready to leave for work. We kiss and say good-bye. I move to the window and wave as she drives away. I'm on my own until 10:00 a.m., when Marilyn comes to feed me and do some light housework. Marilyn is a nice lady, and I enjoy having her around. I get to have Marilyn two hours a day, five days a week, thanks to the government. After she leaves, I watch television or work on the computer.

I have an environmental control unit that helps me change the television channels and turn on lights. It also helps me answer the telephone and make phone calls from my chair. We have three doors to the outside that I can open with the environmental control unit, and I always have my briefcase on my lap, just like a lap tray. Kathleen has put Velcro on the bottom of the environmental control unit and attaches it to my briefcase. The government has made all this wonderful technology available. At 2:30 p.m., Ty gets home from school, and Tucker bounces in around 2:45 p.m.

3:00 P.M.

The boys are supposed to work on their homework as soon as they get home, and I'm there to answer questions or just be supportive. Then I watch television until Kathleen gets home from work, anywhere from 6:00 p.m. to 8:30 p.m., depending on how much work she has. As soon as she gets home, she starts dinner. We all sit at the dining room table and eat together. Kathleen feeds me. I tried a universal cuff, but I didn't have the strength or energy to hold the fork. After dinner, the boys and I watch some more television, while Kathleen stretches out on the couch. She usually falls asleep, and who can blame her? She works too hard, not only at the hospital, but also with me. I hate to wake her, but if I don't, I fall asleep in my chair. I try to go to bed between 9:00 and 10:00.

10:00 P.M.

Kathleen gives me my nightly medications and prepares to put me to bed. I pull my chair up to the bed, and Kathleen takes my shirt off. Then she raises the chair seat above the level of the bed, blocks my knees, and pivots me onto the bed. I am now sitting on the edge of the bed. She lifts my legs over onto the bed. I am lying on my back, and she takes my sneakers and AFOs off. She removes the leg bag and hooks it to the side of the bed. She removes my pants and exchanges the leg bag for the overnight drain bag.

Kathleen also does range-of-motion exercises on me almost every day. Basically, she stretches my arms, legs, ankles and wrists. She says that this helps prevent contractures, which occur when your muscles become very tight and stay that way. Once that happens, it is almost impossible to get them back to normal.

She then prepares my nightly shot of Copaxone and gives it to me in the stomach. She covers me, and we kiss good night. If I'm not sleepy, I watch the news or David Letterman, but if I fall asleep, Kathleen will have to wake up to turn the television off.

◆   ◆   ◆

That is my day in a nutshell, unless it's a bath day or a poop day. They're a little different. I know many of you wonder how I can live this way. Well, I don't have a choice. This is my life, and I accept it. I don't like it a whole lot, either, but if it's all you have, you hold on to it. I don't think you ever learn to like the routine, but it does become bearable.

CHAPTER 19
Pike's Peak View

Our house faces directly west. Before the house across the street was built, we had a beautiful view of the summit of Pike's Peak. After all the houses were completed on the block, we could still see the Peak between two rooftops from the front room window. Through the years, the growth of trees has blocked the view. In the fall after the trees have lost their leaves, we can still see a little of the summit.

Every New Year's, members of an organization in town climb the Peak and set off fireworks at midnight. The Add A Man club has been doing this for many years. As the name suggests, each year they add a new member. In order to be that new member, you have to be some kind of bigshot. Can you believe I was never invited to join?

Our Little Colorado Home

I think I've mentioned that when we were building the house, I was already in a manual wheelchair. That was good in the long run, because as my disease progressed, the house was already set up to handle my increasing disabilities.

We have only made a few modifications through the years. Most of the ramps were in place, off the deck in the back and in the garage. But when we first built the house, our realtor told us not to put a ramp going into the front door, because it would show that a disabled person lived in the house. For whatever reasons, we accepted that at the time. But at some point, I decided I wanted to go in and out my own front door. So we had a wooden ramp built out the front door. The fellow who built it did a real nice job. From the street, it looks like a deck.

The original shower stall became impossible for me to negotiate, so we had a roll-in shower installed. Kathleen hates this shower and wishes she had done more research on different types. She hopes someday soon we can have this shower replaced with a better one.

This is something worth mentioning for the sake of other MS patients. As my condition worsened and I had trouble turning doorknobs, Kathleen replaced the knobs with handles. At first, it really helped me open doors, but now, even using the handles has become too difficult.

The sliding glass door to the backyard was getting harder and harder for me to open, but Buddy still had to be let out at least twice a day. The harder the door got to slide, the more often I used my chair to open it. This wasn't a good idea, because my chair broke the seal around the glass, and we got a lot of condensation between the panes. Kathleen and I decided that the door was not keeping the cold out like it used to and we should replace it, which we did through a local company. They were really good at securing the door so I could roll out to the deck without damaging the door. However, the new door was a lot heavier, and I still could not open it. I didn't want to use my chair and take a chance on breaking the new door.

So, there I am, in the house, and I can't let the dog out to do his business. Not to mention that I was trapped inside if there was ever a fire. Kathleen and I knew we needed to do something. She had been talking to her friend, Eric, an occupational therapist who works for a rehabilitation equipment company in town. He suggested that we try to get approval to have automatic door openers installed. Kathleen and I thought that sounded like a great idea.

Eric also explained that there was a unit that would help me not only open doors, but help me with the phone, the lights, and a lot of other things. So, we applied for an environmental control unit. Within a short period of time, we received approval for the new unit and the power doors. Six months later, all the work was completed.

We thought they would just put a door opener on the sliding door we already had. Instead, they put in a whole new door. Kathleen and I jokingly call it the 7-11 door. That's what it looks like, but it works. They installed an opener on the door to the garage, so I can also open the big garage door with the ECU. Now I can be home alone and still get outside for any reason. Another potential crisis was averted.

Do you remember that I said it was important for an MS patient to keep their core temperature within an acceptable range? Our little house in Colorado Springs doesn't have central air, so it's fortunate that only a week or two in the summer ever gets over eighty degrees. Still, we bought a window air conditioner just for those times. When the temperature goes up, I just sit and watch television all day in front of the window unit. We also installed a motorized ceiling fan that cools the living room.

CHAPTER 20
Some Final Thoughts

I would tell any newly diagnosed Multiple Sclerosis patient today that his or her prognosis is not grim at all. Twenty years ago, there wasn't much available as far as treatments went. But now, it seems that every month or so they come up with new things to try.

The medical profession is constantly researching new treatments, and it's my hope that they will find a cure for this disease soon. I've talked about divine intervention, which you certainly cannot count on, and about prayer, which can't hurt and may help keep things in perspective. Praying to be cured is not really the answer, but praying for the strength to get through each day may be.

As long as you listen to your body and search out a qualified doctor with experience treating MS, you should be guided down the right path. I can't tell you to follow whatever advice the doctor gives you, but you need to find a doctor who will manage your disease for you. Hopefully, your doctor will have your best interests at heart.

Depending on your circumstances, other specialists may be required. These may include: a physiatrist, to provide rehabilitative therapy; a neurologist, to manage the basic MS symptoms; a urologist, to control and medicate for bladder infections, kidney stones, and sexual dysfunction; and a good general physician.

Other professionals that may be helpful in managing your symptoms include physical therapists, occupational therapists, speech therapists, and wheelchair seating specialists. It is very helpful to make contact with someone in social services and your insurance carrier to help you with all the paperwork.

My advice to newly diagnosed patients is to get through the denial stage as quickly as possible. If you have been diagnosed, have had an MRI, and have been told by a qualified professional that you have this disease, it's time to believe it. Evaluate your current status and start working toward maintaining it, without getting worse.

You certainly have the right to be angry. Get your anger out. Yell, scream, and cry until the cows come home. Then concentrate on yourself and the disease. I'm not suggesting that you accept the disease submissively, but that you concentrate on your condition.

Denial. Anger. Acceptance. It can take a long time to get through all three of these stages. I don't think that anyone truly enters the acceptance stage easily. No matter what stage you feel you are in, you should always keep hope in your heart, for it is hope that keeps us all going.

I have shared my past and my present, not so you will do the same things I did, but rather to inform and entertain you and, just maybe, reassure you that you are not alone. I can only hope you'll develop the capacity to laugh, or even cry, about your experiences. Kathleen and I sure have laughed a lot over the past twenty years, and I know that has helped our situation greatly.

When I was young, I didn't think much about time. There was always tomorrow or sometime in the future. I didn't make plans for anything that might happen more than a month into the future. My thinking was that if it was a long ways off, I would deal with it then. I remember starting college and thinking that four years was a lifetime away. If something needed to be done, it could be done on my own time.

Now, time for me is geared around other people's whims. Because of my disabilities, things have really done an about—face. I am virtually dependent on everyone. Time is important, but it is not mine. For instance, in the morning on my back in bed, I whistle for Kathleen to help me. I whistle because I cannot yell as loud as I can whistle. I certainly do not think that Kathleen is some sort of dog. It is just the most efficient way to get her attention. Sometimes she is downstairs or taking a shower, and I have to wait. Sometimes she hears me and says, "Just a minute," and I wait.

Once I am in my chair, I do get some of my time back. When I need help to do something, I can yell for the kids if they are home. I sometimes get, "I'll be there in a minute." It often seems that the minute turns into many minutes.

I've always had a problem with depending on other people. Once you become dependent, that notion won't work. It sure brings home the reality of it all.

I am now concerned with the time when I won't be around. I don't dwell on it; I just think about it. When I was young, insurance wasn't important to me. I might have sold it and truly believed the customers needed it, but I always felt that having life insurance was like betting against yourself.

Getting insurance now would be very expensive, if I could get it at all. Term insurance is like paying until something happens. It is money thrown away for the time nothing happens. In other words, there is no cash value. Kathleen does carry term insurance on me through her employer. Hopefully, that will be sufficient.

Each new healthcare emergency brings about a better understanding of the inevitability of this disease. At these times, if I'm not the one making jokes, it's Kathleen who says just the right thing to get us through another stressful situation. We do have times when we are serious. Our life is not all fun and games.

There are times when I have to think about my body, this disease, and what is going to happen. I try not to dwell on it, and I try to concentrate on more pleasant things. I know Kathleen worries, but, like I've always said, it will come out in the laundry. It's funny, but most things I say that about do work out in the long run. When I first met Kathleen, she would worry over the littlest thing. I started saying my laundry thing, and I think she realized things do work out for the best. Have faith!

Not long ago, my friend Peggy sent me this via email: <u>Whatever God will bring you to, God will bring you through.</u> That kind of says it all.

I met Peggy when I was working at the mall. We hit it off immediately. She was easy to talk to and was married, with two young girls. She eventually started to help me in the store. Peggy is very spiritual, and knows and feels a lot. She knew that she had been adopted, but never wanted to seek out her birth mother. During the time she was working for me, she decided she wanted to know who her real mother was. Within two weeks, she knew who and where her mother was. It was exciting to be around her while all this was developing.

Peggy could see things before they happened. One day she came into the store crying. I asked her what was wrong, and she said that she had had a vision of me walking. She described the scene. It was night-time, and Kathleen and I and Peggy and her husband were walking in a parking lot, coming from a sports bar. She described what we were wearing.

At the time, we were talking about opening the sports bar, but I was still in the store. As time went by and we opened the sports bar, I couldn't wait to see if her vision would come true. Unfortunately, nothing ever happened. I try to keep in touch with her. She is a good friend.

◆   ◆   ◆

With new-fangled computers and the internet, getting information about multiple sclerosis is much easier than ever before. There are many websites that are geared to MS. The one I like is called MS watch. It is very informative and will keep you aware of any new developments.

◆   ◆   ◆

As I said before, if you are not handicapped or disabled, please try to stay aware of things around you that could be a barrier for someone in a wheelchair, on crutches, or using a walker.

I'm always amazed when people, even those who are close to me, are oblivious to certain situations. Recently, a relative was visiting our house and had pulled into the driveway behind another car, and his car was sticking out over the sidewalk. When it was brought to his attention, he said people in his neighborhood parked that way all the time. He did eventually move his car to make the sidewalk accessible. It really bothered me to have a car parked in front of my own home that would not only have limited wheelchair access to the sidewalk, but also would have forced a bicycle or baby carriage into the street.

We all need to consider the needs of others. That shouldn't be asking too much. Those of us who are disabled must continue to use our voice to express our special needs. As I've said, I watch my share of television, and one of my favorite channels is the Travel Channel. We get a lot of different channels on cable, but I can wander all over the world just by watching this channel.

A couple of the shows are very interesting. One features exotic islands. Lovely Hunter Reno takes the viewers to all these great islands and gives us a tour. The second show spotlights great hotels. On this one, Samantha Brown takes us to beautiful hotels and shows would-be travelers the amenities. I think these shows should include information about facilities available for disabled people. In my opinion, they are really missing the boat by not including this type of information. I recently heard that AARP estimates there are forty million people who are elderly or disabled. None of us may have a lot of money individually, but if you put us all together, there are some bucks out there.

I've been fortunate to do some traveling in the States, and it's all been by van. I have stayed in some very fine motels and hotels. It's surprising what some businesses think it takes to make a room accessible to the handicapped. The hospitality industry puts up a couple of grab bars in the bathroom and calls the room handicapped-accessible. How little they know. Some motel owners say they've been exempted from the law because they have been grandfathered in. Remodeling a room to make it handicapped-accessible may cost a few bucks, but in the long run, it should benefit the business. The room could still be rented to a non-handicapped person.

One of the best accessible rooms I ever saw was in an old hotel in Boston. These people had it together and made a great room in a real old hotel, except that the room was on the fourth floor. If there is ever a fire, they always tell you not to use the elevator. My chair, with me in it, weighs 520 pounds. It would take at least three large men to carry it down the stairs. How would you feel about leaving a $25,000 chair behind in a burning building? I guess in the long run I would leave the wheelchair, against my better judgment. After a while, your wheelchair becomes part of you and serves as your legs, so without it, you're not going anywhere. If there is a fire in a hotel, no one will be coming to look for you. I heard a story about a man in a wheelchair during the twin towers episode who didn't want to leave his wheelchair. He had to be carried out.

Maybe someone should start a new show that would explain to the disabled public what is available, not only at hotels and motels, but on ships and airlines, too. There used to be a local wheelchair rep who did a lot of traveling for the VA. He used to publish the do's and don't's of traveling with a wheelchair, but I haven't seen anything by him in a long while.

A friend of mine owned a rehab equipment store, and I used to see what the airlines did to power wheelchairs. It wasn't pretty. As a matter of fact, carriers used to suggest you crate up your chair before you put it on a plane. It would be wise to check before you plan to fly.

The second problem you face when you travel with a power wheelchair is what you're going to do once you get to your destination.

Some airports have wheelchair-accessible vans available to take you to your hotel, but not all do. There are agencies that rent vans in most large cities, but they're pretty pricey. These are just a few of the reasons Kathleen and I always drive our van. It may take us a little longer to drive than it would to fly, but it eliminates many of the hassles.

◆　　　◆　　　◆

I would be thrilled to end this story by telling you that the medical field had made great advances and discovered a miracle drug, and that everyone suffering with this disease would soon be completely cured. I would love to tell you that this morning I woke up and was inexplicably healed, and could put this book down and start writing the next one. But I have to be realistic. I am ending this story in the same way I started it, telling the truth, which is that I am neither walking, nor am I moving as well as when I began this book.

◆　　　◆　　　◆

I have shared a lot about my life with you on these pages, but I think you deserve to know more. I have asked Kathleen if she would write down her thoughts and feelings. Her enlightenment is next.

CHAPTER 21
My Kat'leen's Perspective

Life with Van has been quite a learning experience, and I have grown immensely, both personally and professionally, as a result of being in a relationship with him. I was excited for Van when he finally sat down to compose this book, yet skeptical about revealing our life to the public if the book ever went into print. There is not much that I reveal to others about our personal life, and there are many people whom I have known for years who have heard little or nothing about Van's past. His relationships are not anything that either one of us is very proud of, but I believe those experiences are a part of what molded him into the wonderful and caring father and spouse that he is today.

It has become evident to me, in dealing with a wide variety of individuals over the years, that people have a tendency to gain strength from the experiences of others, especially those who are, or who appear to be, less fortunate. Let me explain. There have been many instances in my work as a physical therapist in which the patient that I am treating makes a comment about another patient he has observed, who appears to be in a worse predicament than he is himself. The observing patient will make a comment like, "I thought I had it bad, but look at what he has to deal with. If he can do it, so can I." I think Van's intention in writing this book is to try to help those in similar situations gain strength from him through his experiences. That is my intention as well, but from a slightly different perspective.

I was in my early twenties, just out of college, and had never been married. I had put all personal wants, needs, and pleasures on hold in order to realize my dream of becoming a physical therapist, and now, barely into my first job, I had met a man who would change my life forever. His name was Van.

As you may have guessed, my decision to marry Van was a difficult one, and I spent well over two years trying to determine the path I should take. After all, he had been married before, and, of even more concern to me, he had a progressive, debilitating disease. The causes and prognosis were unknown, and the treatments were limited. I had many discussions with my parents, and many conversations with God, other family members, friends and, yes, even a counselor.

My parents did a phenomenal job of supporting me throughout my life, including this period of indecision. They always wanted what's best for me, and they had grave concerns that I would take on too much. "You will go to work all day, and then you will come home and work some more," my father said. My dad was a doctor, and he asked me if I knew all of the things that could go wrong with Van because of the MS. I could verbalize it at the time, but, looking back, I know I didn't do a good job of internalizing it. After all, I was young and fresh, with a lot of energy, and I felt I could handle anything.

There was also the issue of Van's previous marriages. The Catholic faith, my faith, does not recognize divorce without an annulment. I have struggled with this issue and continue to question where I sit with God in this matter.

My parents were never overbearing and, ultimately, I knew the decision was my own. It wasn't that my parents didn't care for Van, but they wanted the best possible life for me. Knowing they were probably right, I tried to break it off with Van. But it was difficult for me, for whatever reason, and I continued to see him. There is not any one event I can remember that triggered my decision to marry him, but at one point, I just told Van to take the diamond he had given me months earlier and place it in a setting which I had picked out.

The plans and preparations leading up to our wedding were pretty ordinary. I had a few regrets regarding that day. I wasn't being married in the Catholic Church, and I could not have my sister, Lynne, play the organ for my ceremony. I had always planned that she would play at my wedding, but no one was allowed to touch the pipe organ in the Methodist church we had chosen except the church's organist. Before I walked down the aisle on Dad's arm, Mom said, "You're really going to do it, aren't you?" This was a difficult choice for me, but I knew she loved me and was only looking after my interests.

Van's MS was pretty stable early in our marriage, and we enjoyed getting out and doing things together. We didn't let the disease or the disability interfere with our lives. There were times I was a little disappointed, when I thought the focus should have been on me, but we were forced to focus on Van's needs. The most difficult time for me was when I had a newborn, and Van wound up in the hospital with an exacerbation. I had little time to recover, and less time to enjoy our new son. Early on, these complications were few and far between, but they have increased in both number and frequency as the disease progresses.

My experiences with Van and the disease progression helped me grow immensely as a young physical therapist (P.T.). Van and I learned the ropes together, and there were many life experiences and lessons about disability that I could never have learned from any book. It is my feeling that I have become a better P.T. and am able to connect better with my patients, and especially their families, because of what I have gone through with my own husband.

There were many struggles, conflicts, and feelings of guilt I faced as I attempted to define my role as a full-time employee, wife, mother, and as the progressive caregiver of my spouse. Van was pretty self-sufficient early in our relationship, and I did the usual juggling that a mother does with sports and other extracurricular activities. The kids seemed normal and happy, and I always felt that they would handle the MS well, since they had only known their dad in a wheelchair. Little did I realize what a source of guilt this would become for me later. Although the kids love their father, they, like me, miss the physical part of him. I know Van misses it, too. I have done my best to fill that void with the boys. It's a good thing that I'm a tomboy at heart, who can enjoy outdoor activities with them.

As a physical therapist, it is ingrained in me that a person with a disability should follow all of the medical instructions given, in order to live a life with as few difficulties as possible. I learned quickly that this Pollyanna-type approach is not how life works, but it was, and continues to be, a huge struggle for me. After all, I see the worst of the worst at the hospital, and I know the potential catastrophes that non-compliance can cause.

It is only appropriate at this point to discuss the disease process, and the potential sequelae (per Stedman's dictionary: the morbid condition following as a consequence of a disease). As mentioned earlier in Van's portion of the book, multiple sclerosis is an auto-immune disease that attacks the central nervous system, including the brain and the spinal cord. The course of the disease is different for each individual, and for each type, and there are many types. Common problems are double vision or other visual disturbances, including blindness, balance deficits, sensory deficits, tremor, fatigue, and weakness. More severe conditions include cognitive and emotional problems, bowel and bladder issues, sexual dysfunction, paralysis, spasticity (abnormal increase in muscle tone), and swallowing problems. Some of these symptoms, if not managed well, can lead to additional, life-threatening illnesses, including pneumonia, sepsis, blood clots with the potential for pulmonary emboli (blood clots in the lung), and contractures (which are only life threatening in that they can lead to positioning and hygiene problems, which, in turn, can lead to pressure sores and possible sepsis, as well as collapse in the rib region, limiting breathing capacity).

"I don't want to." You can imagine the turmoil going on in my head when I hear these words from Van. The little mishap that Van alluded to earlier in this book in which I turned his chair off, pushed him back into the house, and put him to bed against his will, and our discussions that followed, have caused me to only do as he will allow, regardless of what I know should be done to keep him in optimal health. There is a resentfulness that I feel when I have to deal with the consequences of his poor decisions. I have told him many times that when he makes a decision for himself, he has also made a decision for me, whether I like it or not.

There are many things that should be done on a regular basis to maintain optimal health, and the list becomes longer as the disease progresses. Diet and fluid intake are essential, and exercise, at an appropriate level, is a must. Medical management of the disease is crucial, as there are many different medications and therapies available to keep some of the symptoms at bay and to assure optimal function. A good support system for the person with MS, as well as for the family, makes all the difference.

In spite of the best care, there is an element of frustration when the disease continues to take its toll. Van's loss of independence has been my loss as well, and this is where survival skills are oh-so-crucial. We have learned to help each other out. We talk a lot, and Van's attitude has made all the difference. He's not a complainer, and most of the time I have to drag information out of him when I see that he is not feeling well. As Van mentioned earlier, he has always told me that things will come out in the laundry, and they generally do. One other thing that Van does that makes all the difference for me, is that he never takes my care of him for granted, and he thanks me for what I do for him. He also acknowledges that my job is not an easy one, and that if he could lift my burden, he would.

There are many things that I do that help me to survive. I realize that frame of mind and attitude make all the difference. This verse by Charles Swindoll has carried me far:

> The longer I live, the more I realize the impact
> Of attitude on life. Attitude, to me is more
> Important than the past, than education, than
> Money, than circumstances, than failures, than
> Successes, than what other people think or say

Or do. It is more important than appearance,
Giftedness, or skill. It will make or break a
Company…a church…a home. The remarkable thing
Is we have a choice every day regarding the
Attitude we will embrace for that day. We can-
Not change our past…we cannot change the fact
That people will act in a certain way. We can-
Not change the inevitable. The only thing we
Can do is play on the one string we have, and
That is our attitude. I am convinced that life
Is 10% what happens to me and 90% how I react to
It. And so it is with you…We are in charge of
Our Attitudes! Winners make commitments. Losers
Make promises.

I can't say that I don't have down times, or that I don't struggle, but recognition of having a poor frame of mind is the first step in correcting it. I have come to the conclusion that when my attitude is wrong, everything is wrong. Thoughts of failure with Van, the kids, and my work creep in and cause a downhill progression from bad to worse. It is so important to keep a positive attitude. This can be difficult when fatigue is heavy upon you. This all circles back, I have found, to taking care of yourself, even if other areas of your life have to suffer. I have had to learn this again and again the hard way, since my subconscious attitude has always been that I must be everything for everyone.

Taking care of myself, as a survival skill, is difficult in the midst of excessive fatigue and an overloaded schedule. At times, Van really has to help me figure out what is my highest priority, because I feel that everything on my To Do list belongs at the top. For me, getting enough sleep is crucial, and proper diet and exercise make all the difference in my attitude.

There are many things that I gain strength from, and my faith in God is number one on my list. Even though my spirituality has waxed and waned through all of this, I have always found strength in the following:

FOOTPRINTS IN THE SAND

One night I had a dream. I was walking along
The beach with the Lord, and across the skies
Flashed scenes from my life. In each scene I
Noticed two sets of footprints in the sand.
One was mine, and one was the Lord's. When the
Last scene of my life appeared before me, I
Looked back at the footprints in the sand, and,
To my surprise, I noticed that many times along
The path of my life there was only one set of
Footprints. And I noticed that it was at the
Lowest and saddest times in my life. I asked
The Lord about it: "Lord, you said that once I
Decided to follow you, you would walk with me
All the way. But I notice that during the most
Troublesome times in my life there is only one
Set of footprints. I don't understand why you
Left my side when I needed you most." The Lord
Said: "My precious child, I never left you
During your time of trial. Where you see only
One set of footprints, I was carrying you.

My family has been a major source of strength for me, along with God and Van. My parents gave me a good, solid foundation. They set an excellent example, not so much through their words as through their lifestyle and their actions. They were hard workers, and I often gain strength by reflecting on how they made marriage, work, and caring for a multitude of children look so easy. They had to be chronically tired, and yet they carried on with a sense of calmness, without complaint.

My brothers and sisters have also been a source of strength for me. Each of them has touched me in one way or another, and to explain in detail would be a book in itself. Needless to say, we are a close family, and my siblings are always there for me when times get tough.

Our children, Ty and Tucker, are an inspiration for me as well. Having children is always a reason to get up in the morning, but these children are special. Although they admit that they would like their father to be well, they don't dwell on his illness. They lighten our tense situations, and they support me when I'm down. They offer comfort just by recognizing that things in our life are more difficult than most, and by showing concern.

I also draw strength from my coworkers. On a regular basis, they ask me how Van is doing. In times of crisis, my coworkers have pulled together to provide overwhelming support through kind words, financial assistance, meals, and physical help. The management at work has always accommodated our situation, allowing me to come and go as needed, in order to assure Van's needs are met. I have truly been blessed.

There is a silent group of people, some I have met and some who I only know exist, who also give me strength. I meet many of them on a regular basis through my work in the hospital. They struggle on a daily basis, just as we do. The elderly in particular, in spite of their physical difficulties, have an overwhelming drive to survive. Oftentimes, the patient's spouse has ailments of his or her own, which compound the problem. There are others I've met who are living in the same situation, but who have more children and do not have the support of their ill spouse. Whenever I see someone trapped like that, it inspires me to try harder, and I remind myself every day that if they can do it, so can I.

Finally, I think of the poor who are exhausted from working several jobs, who are hanging by a thread. They continue to trudge on, one day after another. At least I have the financial stability and the knowledge to care for Van. Again, I am grateful for what I have, and for the tools I possess in order to see this thing through.

To sum it up, it is important to identify the resources you can draw on to gain strength in order to continue to survive a chronic illness, not only for the family member who is ill, but also for everyone else who is taken along for the ride. It is also vitally important to keep a positive attitude and to maintain optimal health. Your support system is critical for your survival, and it is crucial that those family members, friends, and coworkers do not get burned out by repetitive complaints that they have no control over. Your thoughts can't be clouded by what may come, but instead should be consumed by doing what's necessary for your immediate survival.

In spite of many misfortunes in Van's life, I believe that he was inspired to write this book for therapeutic reasons, both for himself and for others who have had similar experiences. He has experienced many failed relationships, in addition to the multiple losses that have resulted from an unrelenting, chronic illness. And yet, his attitude and humor have made all the difference in the outcome, both for himself and for our family. Because of this man, I have become a better person.

AFTERWORD

[total devastation]

The word devastation does not even come close to the feeling when you lose a immediate member of the family. On June 21,2005, we lost our youngest son, Tucker, my inspiration for writing this manuscript.

Tucker was 14 years old, 5 ft. 8 in tall and 180 pounds. He was to enter his first year in high school come August. Tucker was as strong as a bull and a good swimmer.

He left the house about 12:30 that day with his friend Kevin and Kevin's little brother Mark. They were heading to 7-11. This was something they did most days. Early in the afternoon we had a tremendous thunderstorm with hail. As I watched the storm I was thinking when Tucker got home I would tell him it was quite a frog choker. I did receive a call from Tucker saying he was with Kevin. I assumed he was at Kevin's house.

Kathleen got home late that evening and asked were Tucker was. I told her he was with Kevin. It was after dinner time and Tucker should be home or at least called. He had not yet. Assuming Tucker was at Kevin's house, Kathleen went to pick him up. Tucker and Kevin were not home. Kevin's brother Mark was home. They had dropped him off and went back out.

This was not like Tucker. So, Kathleen started frantically look for Tucker. She actually got zero help from the local authorities after several attempts to gain their help. After searching all night with no success. In the morning Kathleen and Ty started searching again. Because of the storm they began looking in the drainage ditches. About midday they said a small prayer and within the next few minutes they found Tucker. The coroner's report said that he had drowned.

Tucker knew about flash floods and all about the ditches. We do not known how or why they were in the ditches. They found Kevin six and one half miles from where Tucker was found.

It has been extremely difficult to comprehend that Tucker is gone. Things will never be the same again. This happens to other families not ours. Kathleen's family were at the house almost immediately. Kathleen's mother and big sister, Lynne, stayed with us for a month. With out them I don't think we would have made it. My older boys, Kane and Mark, were here and they help me a lot. We love Tucker and will always miss him.

His brother Ty has done some memorials for his little brother. They were very well done and he did a great job. We found that a lot of people love Tucker too.

978-0-595-38133-3
0-595-38133-2